nocturnal

SUE JOHANSON AND THE SUNDAY NIGHT SEX SHOW

admissions

RJ GULLIVER with JULIE SMITH

Includes bonus chapter by Sue Johanson

NATIONAL LIBRARY OF CANADA CATALOGUING IN PUBLICATION DATA

Gulliver, R. J. (Randall J.)
Nocturnal admissions : Sue Johanson and the Sunday Night Sex Show

ISBN 1-55022-502-2

1. Johanson, Sue 2. Sunday night sex show (Television program)
3. Sex instruction — Canada. I. Smith, Julie
II. Johanson, Sue III. Title.

PN1992.77.S85G84 2002   613.9'071   C2001-904075-X

Cover and text design by Tania Craan
Front and back cover photos by Richard Beland
All interior photos copyright RJ Gulliver unless otherwise noted
Layout by Mary Bowness

Printed by Transcontinental

Distributed in Canada by
General Distribution Services
325 Humber College Blvd.
Toronto, ON M9W 7C3

Published by ECW PRESS
2120 Queen Street East, Suite 200
Toronto, ON M4E 1E2
ecwpress.com

This book is set in Garamond.

PRINTED AND BOUND IN CANADA

The publication of Nocturnal Admissions has been generously supported by the
Canada Council, the Ontario Arts Council and the Government of Canada
through the Book Publishing Industry Development Program. Canada

The *Sunday Night Sex Show* would like to give a big, fat, tumescent "Thank you!" to the many talented people who have worked on the show over the years. We're sorry if we missed anyone. We were drinking.

Thanks to

Chris Priess	Liz Harding
Rob Bloye	Stacey White
Terry McCarthy	Oliver Weedon
Cathy Johnson	Bill Ferguson
Jason Whyte	Sean Breaugh
Drew Burchett	Frances Bartlett
Derrick Banner	Priya Rao
Lynda Debono	Germaine Wilson
Ali Miraliakbari	Sheldon Wilson
Sana Natur	Seann Harding
Jen Corrigan	Adrian Hepes
Gina Smoke	Stephen Oldfield
Scott Forsyth	Mike Mills
Barb Walld	Arthur Reimel
Susan Millican	Dave Ryan
Shanda Deziel	Terry McAlpine
Jamie Swain	Stephanie Dunthorne
Harvey Heidemann	Tracey Shaw
John Sheppard	Stacey Papagiannis
Kryst Budziak	Dean Bauman
Ivan Kosir	Marnie Starkman
Dwayne Rowe	Erin Sproule
Liisa Robbins	Susan Millican

table
of contents

The Inevitable Disclaimer

Behind the scenes, television workers swear a lot. It's not because they are stupid or inarticulate. (Some would dispute this.) It's because they are in a job that requires a public presentation of absolute propriety — a façade of unrelenting cheeriness and perpetual harmony, where no mortal is ever flustered or picks his or her nose, and where swear words, like tax reforms, are mere shadows of an alternate universe. So, when the cameras aren't rolling, all that pent-up frustration caused by frozen smiles, itchy bums, and plugged noses comes spilling out. It's not a pretty sight. Swearing is a traditional trait of the television industry, much like tattoos are for sailors. (Of course, they swear a lot, too, but that's because getting a tattoo probably hurts like hell.)

Now, bank tellers operate under the same constraints of propriety, but somehow you can't imagine them saying, "Not another *fucking* money order," or "Bounce that cheque up your ass, you *prick!*" Maybe they do when we're not around, but I've never heard it.

Here's my point: this book will have plenty of swearing in it. Be warned. If you're offended by foul language and frank sexual discussions, there's a lovely copy of *My Life as a Bank Teller* just down the aisle from here. I'm sure there's no swearing in it, and it probably contains some really fascinating information about safety deposit boxes.

"Auto Jill"

The four of us stared at the device that Sue Johanson had plunked on the granite table-top with a mixture of incredulity and revulsion, the same sort of look you'd reserve for a dinner host who had just offered you a chocolate-covered fish head.

It was called "Auto Jill."

Technically, it was a masturbation device for men that plugged into the cigarette lighter of a car. It was supposed to represent a vagina in that it had a hole in it. But it was immediately clear that the designers of "Auto Jill" had never actually seen a vagina and had only heard rumours about penises. The hard, plastic device was shaped like a miniature leg of mutton, about eight inches long, with a variable speed-control at the narrow end. It was veined all over with what we assumed was the molded plastic equivalent of pubic hair. The hole seemed far too small to accommodate the average penis. In fact, you would be leery of sticking a pencil in there, let alone your dick.

During his lifetime, the average male will ejaculate 18 quarts of semen containing a half trillion sperm.

"Randy, I want you to take this and try it out," Sue said, averting her eyes in order to avoid an attack of the giggles.

The rest of the production staff — Julie, Frances, and Priya — squirmed in their chairs, checking to make sure that they lacked the required genitals. I suddenly developed eunuch-envy.

In the context of the *Sunday Night Sex Show* production meeting, this was not an unusual request. Crew members often sacrificed their personal time — selflessly subjecting their nether regions to the whims of mad sex inventors — to test the limits of latex, silicone, and AA batteries in order to protect the general populace from potential erotic fatalities. We're sort of the Toy Safety Council for adults. But, "Auto Jill" was going too far. Luckily, I had an out.

"Sue, I'd love to, but I don't have a lighter in my car." Yes, the Japanese — in a smug fit of political correctness — had eliminated lighters and ashtrays from current models of Subaru. Those evil accessories now come as an option: Subaru will kindly aid and abet your Certain Doom for an additional $43. Of course, that was the price *before* "Auto Jill" arrived on the market. The extra power requirements of mobile mastur-bation will undoubtedly lead to a price increase.

Being the director of the show confers a certain set of responsibilities, and one of those is to avoid odious tasks.

"Here. I'll ask one of the guys on the crew to try it out."

Off I went, searching for a suitable sucker who would bravely risk his lineage for the benefit of all Canadian males.

SkyDome is big. I mean, *really* big.

It's so big that you could fit one of the minor pyramids in there and still have room left over for Indy camel racing. On one occasion, they had 48 fully inflated hot-air balloons inside, with the roof closed, which seems kind of pointless when you think about it. ("And below us on the right, a scenic view of Section H." Passengers: "Aaah.") In fact, SkyDome is so big they even let off fireworks in there, a practice that is generally discouraged in an enclosed space. Fortunately, the hot-air balloons and fireworks display have never been scheduled at the same time, or we would have heard about it.

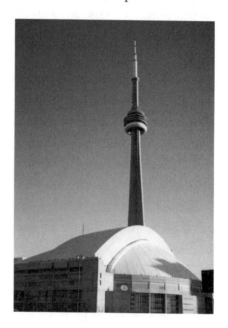

Having never attended an event at SkyDome, I can only assume that the entire audience gets so agitated that they become incontinent, since all 37,000 fixed seats are hosed down after each performance. This process takes eight hours and probably explains why

Two "big" things — SkyDome and the CN Tower

SkyDome smells like a basement full of wet cement.

Of course, it's the home of the Blue Jays, Toronto's erratic baseball team. The largest attendance for a single SkyDome event though was for "Wrestlemania vi," when 67,678 wrestlemaniacs showed up on, appropriately, April Fool's Day, 1990. Extra hosing was required.

Other than its resemblance to a gigantic cervical cap, SkyDome is rarely associated with anything sexual. However, the SkyDome Hotel, which overlooks the playing field, has ended up in the headlines on several occasions when energetic couples made love in their hotel windows, much to the delight of sports fans who suddenly awoke from a baseball-induced stupor and cheered. Hosing has now been extended to the hotel.

So, why ramble on about SkyDome, other than this being the ideal opportunity to mock something really big and stupid? Because SkyDome is not only the home of sports spectacles and entertainment extravaganzas, it's also the home of the *Sunday Night Sex Show*.

Most people are surprised to discover that fact. Viewers tend to think we do the show in an underground bunker near the Swedish Erotica factory. It's not something we've publicized until now. We try to keep it quiet because television equipment is very expensive and does not respond well to gushing water. Also, you never know when the pope might dodder on by to say a public Mass, and we wouldn't want to taint the location. God knows that sex and organized religion have been at odds for centuries, although some would argue that one was invented by God and the other by Man.

The outer walls of SkyDome contain a labyrinth of endless, curved corridors and closed doors. Most doors open to Skyboxes, which are private suites that overlook the playing field below. Some doors lead to food preparation areas and ample beer supplies (more on that later). And a couple of doors lead to Dome Productions, which is where the show originates.

Dome Productions occupies two floors, spread out in a narrow band along one side of the building. The first floor houses an editing suite, a videotape area, the transmission area, and a small bar facility (hey, this was built for jocks). Most of the activity takes place on the second level, with its small studio, make-up room, control room, audio room, and boardroom. That's where I set out from, "Auto Jill" in hand.

I decide to approach one of the "Honorary Originals," a member of the stalwart group that returns week after week.

Now, this may not seem extraordinary, but in the world of freelance television, it is unheard of. The words "loyalty" and "freelancers" are never found in the same sentence. The *Sunday Night Sex Show* is produced by the "Original Seven," who were with the show since it began in 1996, and the "Honorary Originals," who joined the production in the second and third seasons and have become permanent members of the family. They've moved with the show through three different facilities. These are independent television workers — private contractors who give up their families, their leisure, and their evenings every Sunday night, 30 times a year. Often, they have a variety of other bookings early the next morning, but they persevere with the *Sunday Night Sex Show* until after midnight. This is *not* your average group of indifferent freelancers. I corner Dwayne Rowe in the audio room.

"Dwayne, have you got a lighter in your truck?"

"Yup." He's sitting at the audio console with his back to

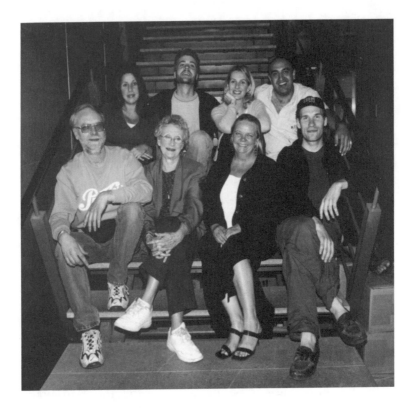

*"Originals" and "Honoraries": (Back row) Sana Natur, Derrick Banner,
Liisa Robbins, Ali Miraliakbari; (Front row) RJ Gulliver, Sue Johanson,
Julie Smith, Dwayne Rowe. Where's Germain?*

me, tweaking the EQ on the show's music playback. "Why? Do
you need a light?"

Dwayne is forever the gentleman, a good-looking guy in
his mid-30s. He's my closest ally in the Control Room. We
work in tandem: I direct the cameras and he mixes the audio,
pictures, and words.

"Well, not exactly. I need a vehicle with a lighter. Sue wants

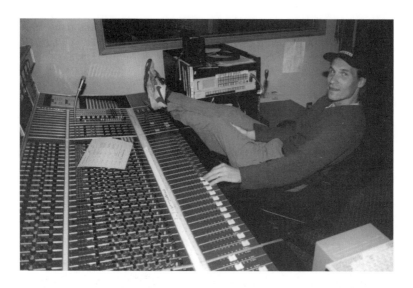

Dwayne works his butt off in the Audio Room.

someone to try out this sex device and it plugs into a car cigarette lighter."

This grabs his attention. He whirls in his chair and stands
to examine it, like he would any new piece of gear. Dwayne
likes gizmos; he was the first person I knew with a digital camera. He started off his career as a cameraman, but there weren't
enough knobs to play with on a studio camera, so he switched
to being a videotape operator. When he was booked on the
Sunday Night Sex Show during our second season, it was to do
tape playback. Upon arriving at the studio, he was informed
that he was also doing audio, although he had never done it in
his life. That's like asking the baggage-handler to pilot the
Concorde. The technical producer at the time reassured him

that this would not be a problem, since the program only had two audio sources: the host and the phone calls. Unfortunately, he failed to mention other factors such as mixing the music in and out, adding audio disclaimers, providing a feed to radio, monitoring the phone calls, and — oh, yeah — the show is live. Dwayne had tackled all that and pulled it off, so I figured he could handle "Auto Jill."

He's got his finger in the rubbery hole. "You mean you're supposed to stick your dick in there while you're driving?" He winces.

Over the course of the show's six seasons, Dwayne has expanded his skills from audio mixer to technical director — which is switching cameras for broadcast as well as overseeing the technical staff and elements — and has even handled directing. On this show, he is completely over-qualified in the audio position, but his loyalty to Sue and the crew brings him back every Sunday night.

"No. It says on the box, 'Do not use while driving.'" I stifle a laugh, trying to present this as rationally as possible under the circumstances. "I guess you could try it out in your garage at home."

"Noooo," he says slowly, "I don't think so." He's shaking his head as he hands it back to me, smiling. "My truck is downstairs in the parking garage. Why don't *you* go down there right now and try it?"

Now that's a terrible thought, getting caught in SkyDome's parking garage, jerking off in someone else's vehicle. I'd get hosed for sure.

"Oh, that's okay, thanks. I'll see if somebody else will check it out."

I leave the audio room and head for the studio down the hall. I certainly understand Dwayne's reluctance. This could be a painful experience. Besides, Dwayne is a very religious person and "auto" erotica would not be something he'd engage in. Both he and his wife, Christine, are devout Christians and they are raising their two children in the faith. Although he personally disagrees with many of Sue's liberal views, he absolutely believes in the educational aspects of her message. He feels that everyone should have access to sexual information and then it's up to the individual to make his or her own choices. He had made his, and it was *not* to try out "Auto Jill."

♀♂

The corridors at Dome Productions always remind me of *Star Trek*, where characters are forever hurrying down curved hallways, delivering crucial plot points just before they enter the turbo-lift and say, "Bridge." Here, we say, "Squirmy Vagina."

The "Squirmy Vagina" was another wacky sex toy that went horribly wrong. As I recall, it was a roundish, passionate purple, gelatinous blob with a vibrator and a hole in it. You could actually see through it, like a quivering Jell-O salad, except instead of banana slices and walnuts inside, there was encapsulated machinery. Since it was blob-like, it would envelop your penis and heat up from your own frantic thrusts, or so I'm told. I never tried it out, but someone on the crew — who shall remain nameless — did. He cleaned it up and brought it back with a bad rating.

The most popular segment of the *Sunday Night Sex Show* is the "Pleasure Chest." It got started because, during our second season, Sue wanted to do a one-hour special on sex toys. She felt that people were interested in buying toys to spice up their sex lives, but were too embarrassed to track them down and examine them in adult stores. Most sex toys are crap, and expensive crap at that, and the ever thrifty — some might say cheap — Sue convinced producer Julie Smith and me that this would be a worthwhile public service. Julie suggested that we do one toy each episode rather than a complete show, and I came up with the segment title. Sue, an inveterate sewer, found an old sewing basket, lined it herself with red velvet, and *voilà*, the "Pleasure Chest" was born.

At first, we didn't actually give the toys a rating. Sue demonstrated (with her hands, please!) how the device worked and commented on its quality and potential for delivering pleasure. But viewers wanted a rating system, so we came up with "Trash, Treasure, or Try It." Hence, our tester had given the "Squirmy Vagina" a rating of "Trash."

Sue showed it on air, gave it the nasty review it so richly deserved, put it back in the "Pleasure Chest," and that was the last we ever saw of it. The chest was stored in the tape library after the show, and the "Squirmy Vagina" vanished during the week. No one on the crew or employed at Dome Productions admitted to taking it. Consequently, we could only arrive at one conclusion: the "Squirmy Vagina" had escaped on its own. Presently, it is still at large, vibrating away in some dark corner of SkyDome, waiting to pounce on some poor unsuspecting penis flopping by. Every Sunday night, at least once when we pass each other in the corridor, someone will ask, with a note of terror in his or her voice, "Has anyone seen the 'Squirmy Vagina?'"

Hence, I kept a tight leash on "Auto Jill" as I approached the studio.

☿♂

The small make-up room is just outside the studio door — it's the province of the formidable Sana Natur, one of the "Original Seven." When people say, "That woman won't take any shit out of anybody," they are drawing on a collective genetic memory of Sana. The only person on the crew who's tougher is producer Julie Smith, and that includes one camera-man who moonlights as a professional wrestler.

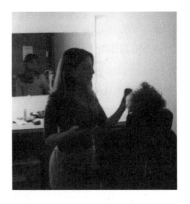

There seems to be a dispro-portionate number of strong women working in television production. It's a tough busi-ness, filled with eccentrics who

Sana and Sue make up.

would be incapable of holding down traditional jobs. Tele-vision people, myself included, are outlaws, outsiders who couldn't tolerate a career in a corporate institution. In earlier centuries, we would have been buccaneers. Hours are long and the politics can be lethal. Thick skin is a prerequisite.

Women in production often find themselves dealing with "talent," which is industry jargon for "self-centred, spoiled brat." Generally, on-air performers have the singular "talent" of being good-looking. There are only two other professions I know of where that's the major requirement — modelling and prostitution.

"Hey, check this out." I show Sana the current albatross.

"Oh my God!" Both her hands rise to her cheeks in mock amazement. "What the hell is that?"

As I explain the subtle mechanics of "Auto Jill" — stick your penis in here; plug it in; don't drive — I'm aware that those boneheads in the sex factory have completely missed the mark if they think they can approximate a woman as striking as Sana with a latex appliance. She is small, amply proportioned, with an exotic, sculpted Mediterranean face. I would imagine that many a man has pined for Sana, but she married a lucky guy named Rob.

"Want to take this home for Rob?" I ask hopefully.

She laughs. "I don't *think* so!"

Aside from being tough, Sana is also fiercely loyal. She would never subject her husband — or anyone else whom she cared about — to this. Sana always operates in extremes. She's as passionate about her friendships as she is about her enmities. That intensity extends to her job — she frequently works seven days a week — and, fortunately, to her considerable sense of humour.

"Sue asked me to try this out but I don't have a lighter in my car. Who do you think I should ask?"

She doesn't miss a beat. "Ask Ali. He's mad."

The studio itself is tiny as far as studios go. It's probably 20 by 30 feet, and that would be a generous guess. This was not a potential location for *Lord of the Rings*.

When we first got to Dome Productions, the studio was even tinier. During our first season there, there was no make-up room. Sue had to change her clothes behind a desk partition in the hallway outside the studio door, and Sana applied her make-up by the light of some "glow-in-the-dark" panties. This may work well for a sportscaster like Don Cherry, whose wardrobe glows in the dark with no additional chemical treatment, but it was decidedly inconvenient for a female host. Dome Productions heeded Julie's protests, added a make-up room, and expanded the studio. Now Sana has an actual make-up mirror and can keep her panties on.

One enters the studio behind the large, curved backdrop that hangs at the back of the set. Viewers have often asked what the pattern on that huge piece of printed vinyl behind Sue is, and here's the low-down: it's strands of DNA. Julie chose it because she liked the look of it and she liked the symbolism. Unfortunately, dozens of innocent people are languishing in Canadian prisons because we're using their DNA for scenery.

Ali Miraliakbari is the black sheep of the "Originals," not because he's unfriendly, but because he's insane. He handles the teleprompter for the show. This involves typing in Sue's script for various segments and the names and locations of phone callers, information he receives on his headset from the Control Room. Initially, his inability to spell was a bit of a hindrance (Caller: Franswa from Cappuscaysing), but he's improved dramatically in that area. He now knows that Kappuscaysing starts with a "K."

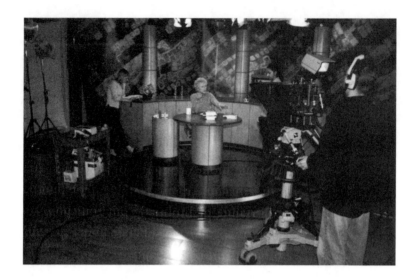

Sue rehearses while Liisa times the script. Derrick's on camera. A stranger's DNA hangs in the background.

During commercial breaks in the broadcast, he tosses out little one-liners from behind his prompter console. More often than not, these gags are snatches from some unknown comedy that's been unfolding in his head alone, leaving everyone else in the studio slightly perplexed and wondering whether psychiatrists make house calls on Sunday evening.

Ah, Ali may be nuts, but he's our nut. What he lacks in spelling acumen is more than compensated for by his boundless enthusiasm. Ali is guaranteed to pick you up when you're feeling down. The teleprompter is not his first love — photography is, and he's a damned good one. Also, when it comes to sexual abandon, Ali cannot be beaten. He's game to take on anything and everything.

"Ali, how's your Fiat running these days?"

"Good," he looks up from his typing. I notice his finger is hovering over "k."

"Does the lighter work?" With Ali's car, this is speculative.

"I think so. Why?"

"We need someone to try this out."

He leaps up from his chair and grabs the box. His sudden interest may have been piqued by the big-haired blonde with boobs busting out of her blouse on the front of the package. As he reads the instructions, he starts cackling hysterically, with the occasional "No way!" thrown in for punctuation. Then he pulls "Auto Jill" out of her box and gives an *"Oooooh"* of revulsion, which was undoubtedly the same noise Sue made when her cat, Hoover, horked up a chipmunk's head. (But that's a whole 'nother story . . .)

"This is disgusting!" he hollers. "How can you fit your cock in there?!"

He's trying to stuff two fingers in to make his point. Forget about shoe-size or hand-width, you can always tell how big a guy's penis is by how many fingers he tries to stuff into a sex toy — present company excepted, of course.

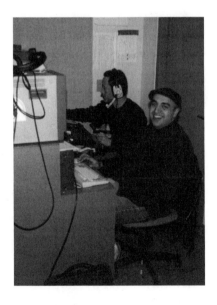

Ali at the teleprompter console. Lighting director Bill Ferguson adjusts light levels.

"And there's a hard plastic ridge in there that would be jabbing the end of your dick!" He's getting very agitated now. Ali is a big bear of a man with a shaved head, and I realize that getting him agitated is probably not a good idea.

"There's *no way* I'm gonna try this out!" He shoves the offending apparatus back into my hands and drops down to his keyboard, determined to ignore me, and it.

So even Ali had said no to "Auto Jill." By now, word was undoubtedly spreading ("Look out for 'A.J.' — Only good for hamsters.") and soon, no one in the downtown core would be willing to try this thing. I hated to do it, but I was going to have to throw myself on the mercy of the sweetest guy on the crew.

♀♂

You know, I'm making it sound like all we do is talk about sex toys the entire evening. Nothing could be further from the truth. We are, after all, television professionals. We also drink coffee and smoke cigarettes.

The show airs live at 11 p.m. Eastern time, but we arrive between 8:00 and 8:30, when every crew member immediately sets to his or her appointed task. After six seasons, we pretty well have this down to a science.

The first order of business for the production staff — those of us with no technical skills beyond being able to navigate the drive-thru at Tim Hortons — is to hunker down for the weekly production meeting. Producer Julie Smith, another "Original," chairs the session.

Julie is also the head of Independent Production for the Women's Television Network, a powerful executive position.

She has a major say in what shows get produced for the network and what shows don't. Prior to her stint with WTN, she spent 18 years as a documentary producer, shepherding crews and reporters around the world, from Africa to Antarctica. The gravity of that journalistic background is clearly evident as we start off the meeting talking about . . . flowers?

Yes, flowers. Sometimes depilatories, but usually flowers. Julie loves to garden, and so does Sue. Spring provides ample opportunity for yapping about nasturtiums, tulips, hyacinths, crocuses, daisies, lilies, and all manner of flora. In the winter, we just talk about Brazilian waxing.

After about 20 minutes of this crucial prep work, we move on to the really important stuff — coffee. We exit the meeting room en masse and head for the control room, hoping that Ivan Kosir, our tape operator and resident coffee-maker, has brewed up a fresh batch. Invigorated, we return to our Very Important Production Meeting.

Aside from the principals — Sue, Julie, and me — there are two other members of the production team: Frances Bartlett and Priya Rao.

Frances is an old friend of mine who did us the favour of filling in as Sue's assistant one night and now won't go away. Like Julie, she is widely travelled, having lived for 10 years in Hong Kong, where she started her own publishing company. She also worked as a cook on a Norwegian cargo ship with seven men, but we won't go into that. She's from Kapuskasing. (Ali, note!)

I met Priya when I was working at CTV, where she was volunteering on a program called *eNOW*. She functions as Sue's assistant, but her real ambition is to be an actor. Priya's family is from India. When she first arrived, she was a very reserved 29-year-old who couldn't tell a dildo from a butt plug. These days, it takes something as outrageous as "Auto Jill" to make her flinch.

Now, I haven't said much about Sue Johanson, the host of the show and the reason we're all here. Sue has such an amazing history that she gets her own chapter later. Dwayne says, "Sue is the glue," and he's absolutely right. Without her, there would be no show. She's like a doting grandmother with a provocative streak: hyperactive, funny, caring, and passionate in her belief that all people have the right to know about sexuality. To Sue, there's no such thing as a stupid question. The fact that she's one of the planet's biggest hams is an added bonus.

A production meeting generally begins in earnest with Sue's feet up on the boardroom table, running shoes notwithstanding. She leans back in her chair, reading the scripted

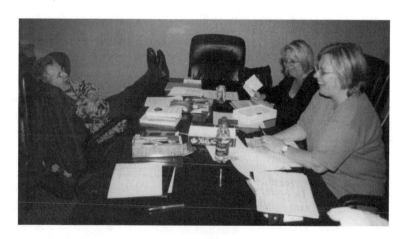

The Very Important Production Meeting: Sue, Julie, and Frances Bartlett give serious consideration to a meaningful topic.

portions of the show out loud. Usually, she writes the script several weeks in advance, and I rewrite portions before the meeting. Frances has a sharp eye for editorial errors and the read-through generally results in a few more minor changes. Sue pulls that evening's sex toy out of her tote bag, and Priya sets off looking for suitable batteries. Sometimes Sue suggests toys or themes for upcoming shows, and sometimes the discussion can get quite heated. (I'll tell you about the blow-up over the Blowup Doll later.) After the meeting, Frances or Priya coordinates the updates with Ali — who has received a floppy with the original script on it — and the rest of us head for the smoking lounge.

Yes, we are bad. Yes, we smoke occasionally. In spite of that, some of us still don't have lighters in our cars. And on that laboured segue . . .

♀♂

There are actually two people who could qualify as "the sweetest guy on the crew" — Germain Wilson and Derrick Banner, our two cameramen. It's a toss up, but since Germain doesn't own a car, that narrows down the choice.

"So Derrick, have you got a lighter in your car?" I've cornered him in the Control Room where he's chugging coffee and scarfing down a sourdough biscuit. (Sue bakes sourdough biscuits for the crew every week.)

"Yes." He pauses, suspicious. Chews a bit. "Why?"

Derrick is also one of the "Originals." He started on the show when he was 21, fresh out of school. He's tall and thin, and, unlike most men, gets more beautiful as he gets older. He's

21

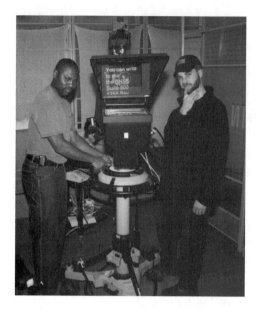

Germain Wilson and Derrick Banner consider the weighty subject of camera ballast.

a very thoughtful, gentle guy — Sana says he was "well raised." During the show's run, Derrick has settled down with a lovely woman named Nicole and her young son. Sue worries about how thin Derrick is. He's the prime target of her biscuits.

"Well, I've got this device to try out and it plugs into a cigarette lighter." I wave it in his face.

"My lighter doesn't work," he says, looking relieved. By now, I'm attracting the attention of everyone else in the Control Room. A groundswell of horror starts to build.

"Well, do you think you might get it fixed this week sometime?"

"OHMYGOD! What *is* that?!" Liisa Robbins is clutching her face in absolute shock, doing a very good impersonation of an Edvard Munch painting.

Liisa — whose parents were presumably so well-off that

they could afford two "i's" — joined the show during its second season as the assistant director, and is one of the "Honorary Originals." She grew up in England, where her school chum, Geri Halliwell, has made quite a name for herself. Liisa's family immigrated to Canada and, until recently, she still lived at home with her parents, who are very strict and conservative. The mere mention of the word "sex" causes jaws to clench and legs to cross. Subsequently, Liisa is the easiest person on the crew to shock, which we all delight in doing.

"Liisa, meet 'Auto Jill.'" I explain its purported capabilities. She looks like she's smelling a fart.

When Liisa first started on the show, she found the calls deeply embarrassing. She was forever blushing. She couldn't believe that people would actually say things like "blowjob" and "eat her out" in a public forum. During the broadcast, she sits right beside me and handles the segment times, adds the

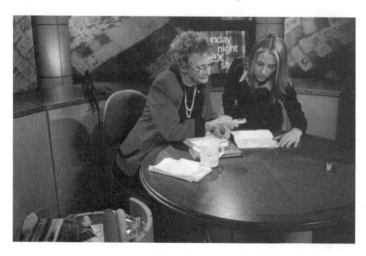

Liisa with Sue going over preshow notes.

text for names, and talks on her headset to Master Control in Winnipeg.

She tentatively pokes a finger into Jill. "Ooooh, how would you *clean* it?!" she asks with her cultured British accent. The Brits — forever practical.

Although her parents know that Liisa works on the show, she regards it as her "secret life." Over the years, she's toughened up a lot and can carry on a very respectable conversation regarding most sexual matters without turning crimson. Once, when relatives were over from England, they watched the show with her parents. Afterwards, she drove home as slowly as she could to avoid the inevitable wisecracks. I expect her at any moment to check her Palm Pilot for scheduled visits.

"Wouldn't it be difficult to fit a penis in there?" she wonders aloud. The sight of this petite blonde with her finger stuck in a mutton-shaped piece of plastic would reduce most colleagues to paroxysms of laughter or lust, but the Control Room takes it in stride.

"How do *you* know how big a penis is?" Liz Harding, the technical director, asks slyly. Liisa, of course, blushes.

Liz is a lively woman with stunning, long red hair who's worked on the show for the last couple of years. She switches the cameras and sources for on-air and sits to my left during the broadcast. It's not unusual, when there's a lull in the action, to find her huddled over her switcher, knitting.

Technical Producer Sheldon Wilson is also sitting in the Control Room, trying to look as inconspicuous as possible. He hasn't been with the show for long and I'm afraid that if I ask him to try "Auto Jill," he'll pass out. As the kerfuffle continues, he scurries out of the room.

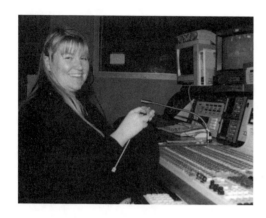

*Liz Harding tackles
the technical
challenge of knitting.*

"Who am I going to get to try this fucking thing out?" I exclaim.

At that moment, Germain Wilson walks into the room.

J.Q. Publik is a rising star on the Canadian independent wrestling circuit, the league that functions as a "farm team" for the big boys such as the WWF.

He currently holds three titles: the Hardcore Wrestling Federation Championship, the Shockwave Wrestling Championship, and the Canadian Independent Wrestling Association Tag-Team Championship. He's a fan favourite and, after a match, T-shirts bearing his logo are a brisk seller. J.Q. is always the first wrestler out of the dressing room, ready to sign autographs, hug excited little kids, and pose for pictures. Often, he'll have a championship belt slung over his shoulder. With his classic, male, inverted A-frame torso of broad shoulders and narrow hips, his waist is too small to hold the belt up.

Fans love him because he's cool and gorgeous: six-foot-two, beautiful black man. He dances on his way to the ring, offering furtive kisses to awestruck ladies crowding the aisles. Of course, he narrowly beats his opponent, who is invariably unscrupulous, then dances back to the shadows, waving his arms in triumph as the crowd stomps their feet in approval.

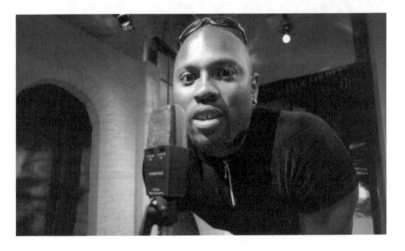

Germain tests a mike. (Photo courtesy Ali Miraliakbari)

In real life, J.Q. Publik is a shy, freelance cameraman named Germain Wilson. He works on the *Sunday Night Sex Show*.

Germain grew up in Scarborough, a suburb of Toronto, with his sister and his mother, Joan, who is an active member of a local evangelical church. When Germain was young he eagerly participated in church goings-on: singing, playing drums, acting in pageants — anything to get on the altar and be seen.

At school, Germain was a quiet, gawky teenager. His report cards would always note, "Germain is a good boy, but he needs to participate more." His paralysing shyness made that impossible. Group discussions were his greatest fear, and still are.

Being on stage was another story. "I'm a big show-off," he says. Germain readily admits to being 100% ham, through and through. He considered going into acting, but instead decided to work in the entertainment industry as a cameraman, and attended Centennial College in Toronto to get his degree.

Germain had always loved professional wrestling. He loved the operatic quality of it, the drama, and the bigger-than-life heroes and villains. When he attended a WWF event at SkyDome in 1997, a stranger handed him a flyer that changed his life. The flyer promoted a small wrestling outfit that was looking for trainee wrestlers and managers. He jumped at the chance.

Germain didn't think he was physically large enough to be a wrestler, so he intended to learn the role of manager, a secondary character in the wrestling passion play. However, he quickly discovered that he could take "bumps" better than anyone else in the course. (A "bump" is wrestling jargon for the oft-used move of kicking both feet straight out and slamming down flat on your back in the ring, an action that one normally and painfully reserves for wet ice.) Germain gave good bump, so he altered his course — he set his sights on becoming a championship wrestler.

Professional wrestling is currently known as "sports entertainment," which, I think, puts it in the same category as any play by Andrew Lloyd Webber. Indeed, Germain sounds like a professional dancer when he admits that, at first, he was terrified that he wouldn't be able to memorize all the moves. But he did, and in three short years, he's gone from the bottom of the slate to the main event.

"The whole point of wrestling is to protect your opponent," he says. Although that's the stated philosophy, it hasn't always worked in his favour. He suffered a concussion once and, in another match, he was badly cut by a garbage can lid. The scar on his forehead is a reminder of that miscalculation.

"It was just an accident. My opponent didn't mean to do it, but the crowd loved it. I still get e-mails about it," he beams.

Germain's wife, Tara, accepts his obsession with resignation, although she has no interest in the sport. His mother, Joan, on the other hand, is dead-set against it. She worries constantly that her son is going to be seriously injured. He understands her maternal fears, but that doesn't stop him. To make matters worse, whenever she attends a match, Germain is inevitably tossed out of the ring, smashing through tables and chairs on his way down. It's all part of the act: he's even named one of his moves in her honour.

"It's called 'Momma's Laundry,'" he explains. "I leap in the air and kick one leg straight out and the other guy runs into it with his throat. It's supposed to be a clothes-line. He bumps and doesn't get back up. And I win." He smiles to himself, reflecting on a recent victory.

Yes, the shy, soft-spoken choirboy from the suburbs is aiming to be a major thumper of men. He knows exactly what he wants — to be in the big leagues, controlling the crowd with the force of his performance, quelling his opponents, and savouring the adulation.

"Why do I love it so much? I think it gives me the same

feelings I had when I used to perform back in the church. It makes people happy, and I love to do that. When I'm signing autographs after a show, people are asking for pictures, and little kids are squealing because they're so excited to meet me, it really makes me feel great. I can make their lives happier and that's the thrill."

♀♂

"What is *that?*" says Germain, spying "Auto Jill" tenuously cradled in Liisa's hands.

He gently takes it from her for a closer examination, and she explains its function, occasionally covering her mouth in embarrassment. A broad grin breaks across his face. He's considering the photographic possibilities.

Like any genuine ham, Germain is more than willing to appear on air, preferably wearing as little as is legally possible. The show takes full advantage of his talents. Sue is forever demonstrating latex body-paint, homemade nipple clamps, and all manner of erotic gewgaws on a semi-naked Germain. Women on the crew, and Sue more than most, openly salivate on these occasions. He has a luscious build and viewers have taken notice. When Sue goes out on lectures now, students yell out, "Where's Germain?" She was doing a radio program in Winnipeg where she was the mystery guest, and listeners had to guess who she was by her "yes" or "no" answers. Finally, a caller asked, in a seductive tone, "Is Germain with you?", and the jig was up. Any other host would feel threatened by sharing the spotlight, but not Sue — she loves it, and she loves Germain.

"I would have asked you if you wanted to try it out," I

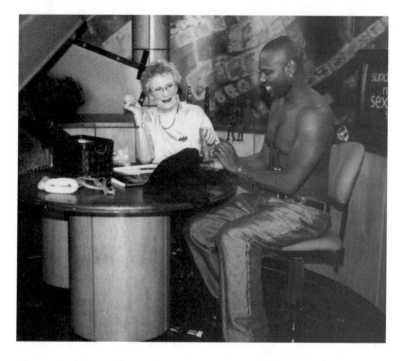

Testing the homemade sex devices on Germain before a show.
Sue is sweating.

apologize, as if I've just denied him a match with Sable, "but you don't have a car. So far, we don't have any takers."

At that moment, Sheldon rushes into the Control Room with engineer du jour Seann Harding in tow. Seann is a sprightly, wiry guy, a biking fanatic, who has probably never even seen first gear. His excitement level generally starts at "10" and ratchets up from there. Nothing gets him going like an engineering challenge, and Sheldon has provided one. Seann's carrying with him a small, primitive-looking device that's a bit larger than a car battery.

"It's a DC converter," he explains, setting it down on the floor by Liisa. "We took it out of the mobile."

Dome Productions owns several mobiles, portable control rooms designed for covering sporting and entertainment events. When not in use, they're parked in the loading dock of SkyDome. Sheldon and Seann had hurried down to that level and retrieved the sophisticated technology that "Jill" demanded.

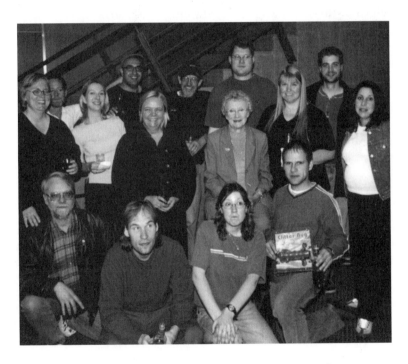

The current family: (Back row from left) Bill Ferguson, Ali Miraliakbari, Harvey Heidemann, Sheldon Wilson, Derrick Banner; (Middle row) Frances Bartlett, Liisa Robbins, Julie Smith, Sue Johanson, Liz Harding, Sana Natur; (Front row) RJ Gulliver, Dwayne Rowe, engineer Jamie Swain, Ivan Kosir. Where's Germain?

By now, the whole gang has gathered in the dimly-lit room — Sue, Julie, Frances, Priya, Dwayne, Sana, Ali, Derrick, Liisa, Liz, Ivan, Sheldon, and Germain. Even Harvey Heidemann, the crusty CBC vet who rides video levels on the show, has made an appearance, lured by coffee, cookies, and commotion. With everyone watching, Seann plugs the toy into the converter, and *voilà*, "Auto Jill" begins to hop.

"Wow! Feel that thing vibrate!" he exclaims. It sure did. We all took turns holding it, poking fingers in, shaking our heads and laughing. We collectively decided that "Auto Jill," unfortunately, vibrated *too* much, and was probably more suitable for mixing cement than for stimulating an orgasm.

"Okay, anyone want to try it out?" I holler over the hubbub. Germain reaches for his fly. "Just kidding!" he shouts back.

Air-time is rapidly approaching, as Liisa reminds us. People start scattering to their posts and Seann unplugs the hapless device and returns it to its box, unsullied by human lust. We turn our attention to broadcasting a live television show.

Alas, poor "Auto Jill" remains a virgin to this day. She's gathering dust in the back of my bedroom closet, pondering her future as a lonely, latex spinster, and nursing her spiteful envy of the "Squirmy Vagina."

You'd be wise to keep your car doors locked.

Luck and Pluck

Unique Lives and Experiences is a Canadian series of lectures given each year by some of the most outstanding women in the world — Dr. Jane Goodall, Erin Brockovich, Shirley MacLaine, Julie Andrews, and Margaret Atwood, to name a few. In the spring of 2000, Sue Johanson was invited to join the prestigious line-up.

She accepted reluctantly. It wasn't the upscale crowd that scared her — God knows, she can talk to anyone, and does. Sue could never be accused of being short on words. What made her jumpy was the subject matter. Sure, she can hold forth for hours about ovarian cysts, micro-penises, blowjobs, and all manner of intimate bodily functions; but this lecture required her to talk about something she never discusses — her personal life.

Like many public personalities, Sue is a very private person. Being in the spotlight tends to increase one's guard over personal thoughts and feelings. With a controversial

"My idea of an aphrodisiac is a naked man doing the dishes wearing nothing but a condom." — Sue Johanson

subject like sex, this effect is even more pronounced. Sue's major concern, as always, is protecting the privacy of her family.

So, when I arrived at posh Roy Thomson Hall in Toronto to hear her speak, I didn't know what to expect.

The hall was packed, completely sold out. Incredibly, there were even people sitting *behind* the stage. The crowd was mostly female, a well-heeled group of the city's elite, ranging from young to not-so-young, and from society matrons to corporate leaders. Here was the top of the food chain. In order to avoid their collective scorn, Sue had to deliver the goods, walking a fine line between sharing her past and protecting her future.

She was politely introduced by her friend, interviewer Jane Hawtin, and then she took to the stage looking more nervous than I had ever seen her. Within two minutes, the nerves had settled and she was working her charm even on this sophisticated bunch. She quickly disarmed them with her self-deprecating one-liners as she prowled the stage looking for all the world like a hen on a mission. She talked of her isolated childhood, her female mentors, her years in the media, and the role of luck in her life. When she got serious, people's eyes clouded with tears. It was an extraordinary, compelling presentation. The standing ovation at the end was prolonged and genuine, and reviews the next day were glowing.

It was a thrill to be there, not just for me but for the entire audience. She had finally given them what they had wanted to know for a very long time — what is Sue Johanson really like?

From her Dickensian childhood to the stage of Roy Thomson Hall, this is how Sue got there.

♀♂

Susan Avis Bayley Powell was born in Toronto during the last millennium. She's touchy about the exact date.

Her father was Wilfrid Bayley Powell of Harpenden, Herfordshire, England. Her

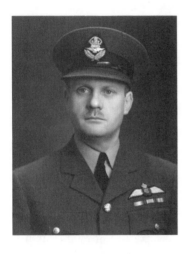

Sue's father, Wilfrid Bayley Powell, was a dashing hero in the war, and to Sue.

mother was Ethel Bell, born in Toronto. They had met on a golf course, a typical meeting place for members of the upper class.

Wilfrid had fought in World War I and had had a spectacular military career. He had enlisted in the British Cavalry, and sustained a leg wound in action. He had been gassed at Vimy Ridge, where he removed his socks, filled them with dirt, pissed on them, and then breathed through them in order to survive the attack. While recovering back in England, he decided he'd had enough of ground warfare.

Flying was the latest weapon in the arsenal of World War I, but it was essentially experimental and chances of survival were low. As soon as he was discharged from the hospital, Wilfrid joined the fledgling Royal Air Force. He ended up piloting a Sopwith Camel. The plane was equipped with bombs at the pilot's feet so that Wilfrid could lob them over the side at German forces below. He also had a pistol for shooting at enemy planes. In his squadron he met a Canadian he liked very much, a fellow named Billy Bishop. Billy suggested that Wilfrid move to Canada after the war, and he seriously considered the suggestion.

When the war ended, Wilfrid was decorated for bravery by the British government, and, like many people who achieve their greatest glory early in life, he never quite recovered from it. While in the cavalry, he had started drinking heavily, and by the war's end, he was an alcoholic. Although he was a war hero, he was unemployable. A move to Canada seemed like a sensible thing to do, and his embarrassed family encouraged his departure.

Ethel Bell was a member of an affluent Irish-Protestant family. Her father, James, was a staunch Orangeman who never failed to march in the annual Orange parade, glowing in his celebratory white flannel suit and white straw hat. James and his wife, Anna, were a dour, hard-working couple who had immigrated to Canada during the Irish Potato Famine. They acquired several properties in Toronto's west end, and Ethel enjoyed a privileged, protected childhood. Ethel was a delicate woman with immaculate skin, green eyes, and long red hair. To her, Wilfrid Powell must have seemed a knight in shining armour — a distinguished, charming British gentleman, a literal hero. They struck up a relationship. His reputation as a drinker and his inability to find steady employment didn't dissuade her. But it certainly affected her family: the Bells hated him. Ethel married Wilfrid against their wishes.

It was a miserable union. They fought constantly. Ethel

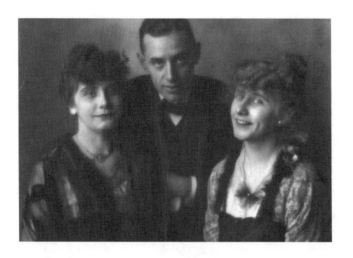

*(From left) Sue's mother, Ethel Bell; real estate
magnate, Cecil White; his wife and Ethel's sister,
the dreaded Aunt Joie.*

ended up moving out and living with her sister, Gladys White
— known as "Joie" (jo-ee) to the family. Joie was also separated from her husband, real estate tycoon Cecil White.

Ethel and Wilfrid tried several times to reconcile. It was
during one of these bouts of forgiveness that their only child,
Susan, was conceived. By the time the baby was born, Ethel
was once again estranged from her husband and had rented a
house on Howland Avenue in downtown Toronto.

Sue doesn't recall her mother ever having a job. They were
supported by her father, who found work as a salesman for the
Gutta-Percha Rubber Company, selling hot-water bottles and
rubber products to stores. The support payments were erratic
and meagre, and Ethel adjusted to a life of genteel poverty.
The one thing Wilfrid did not skimp on was his affection for

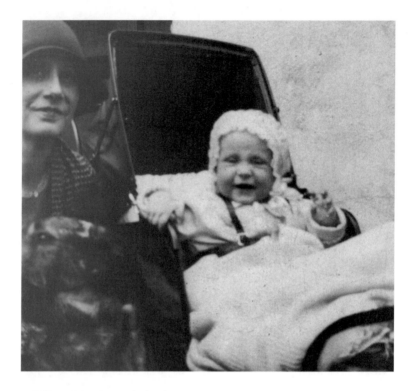

Ethel with her happy baby daughter, Susan Bayley Powell.

his daugher — he adored her, and his love was returned in kind. Unlike the staid Bells, Wilfrid was fun and charming. He would often take Sue out for an afternoon adventure. Occasionally, the outing ended with Wilfrid sitting in a pub while his daughter waited alone outside, swinging on a lamp-post. Once she fell and cut her head on the pavement, and her father had to be hauled out of the pub by a complete stranger to attend to her. Ethel was furious, but Sue defended her dad.

Ethel was an attentive mother, if somewhat distant. Every

Sunday evening, mother and daughter attended family dinner at the Bell residence with Ethel's parents and sister. The tone was always sombre and formal. Grandpa James was virtually silent and the ladies carried the conversation. Children were expected to be seen but not heard, and Sue, their only grandchild, complied.

When she was eight years old, Sue's father lost his sales job and the support payments stopped. Joie offered to take her sister and niece in, and they both moved to her home at 70 Nina Avenue. A year later, Ethel was diagnosed with breast cancer. She died when Sue was 10 years old. Custody of the young girl passed into the hands of the embittered, cold Auntie Joie.

As far as Joie White was concerned, the decline and early death of her beloved sister was solely attributable to one cause — Wilfrid Powell. She hated him with a passion, and because Sue looked like her father, that enmity extended to the child. Auntie Joie would continually put her down with a sarcastic, "You're just like your father." When she didn't do well at school, Joie would remind Sue that she wasn't very bright or very attractive, and that her future prospects were bleak. She was only allowed to see her father once a month for a luncheon date. School was difficult and every report card would note, "Susan would do much better if she learned to apply herself." It was an oppressive existence.

Sue's salvation during this period was a family who lived two doors away, the Files. Ron File was a teacher at Central Tech and his wife, Mabel, was a former teacher herself. They had four children and very little money, but Mabel embraced the motherless girl as though Sue were her own daughter. Sue ate most of her meals there, and returned to her aunt's only to sleep. The

Files were so poor that lunch often consisted merely of ketchup or sugar between two slices of bread. Sue vividly remembers the one glorious summer she went camping for six weeks with the entire File clan. (Her aunt's contribution was a single jar of marmalade.) It was one of the happiest periods of her childhood. Although the Files couldn't provide the amenities available at Auntie Joie's house, they offered what Sue needed the most — the three "A's": approval, acceptance, and appreciation. This was the lesson that would enlighten the rest of her life. Even now, Sue still refers to the late Mabel File as "Mommy File." "They were spectacular to me," she says, her eyes welling up.

There were also two lessons she learned from Auntie Joie, although neither of them were imparted freely. Joie lived an indolent life, supported by her estranged husband, and she read constantly to fill the time. Her niece began to do the same, sometimes reading two or three books a day. Also, Joie was an excellent knitter. Sue was afraid to ask her for instruction, so she got up early one morning, found the needles and some wool, and taught herself how to knit. Eventually, that led to her passion for sewing, one of her favourite pastimes to this day.

When World War II started, Wilfrid enlisted again, this time in the Canadian Army. He was stationed in South Porcupine, Ontario, guarding German prisoners of war. He would write to his daughter regularly, sending her war stamps. Joie would hand her the letter with disdain.

With his previous experience, it wasn't long until Wilfrid joined the Royal Canadian Air Force. He was promptly made wing commander and posted to Brandon, Manitoba, to train new pilots. It was here that he met and fell in love with Bessie Ross.

The Rosses were members of Brandon's elite. They had money and the Ross girls — Bessie and her sister Tina — were well-respected, lively participants of the local social scene. Once again, Wilfrid's good looks and charm had netted a prize catch. They talked of marriage, but he refused to commit to a union without his daughter's approval. Sue was sent for in Toronto, and, at the age of 12, she travelled alone by train to Manitoba, leaving the misery of Auntie Joie behind her. But, it was not the last time that Joie White would play a pivotal role in her life.

♀♂

Bessie Ross became Sue's new mother, and the girl could not have been happier.

Bessie and Tina had inherited their parents' wealth and lived together in the large family home. There was plenty of room for a young girl, and Sue moved right in. Her father was stationed at the base nearby and, every other week, he received a 48-hour pass to return for a visit. During this period, his drinking was confined to the Officers' Mess, so there was little evidence of his alcoholism around his daughter or his new wife.

Bessie absolutely adored Sue and, under her care, the young girl blossomed. Like her father, Sue had naturally curly hair. Both her mother and her aunt had previously let it grow into a long, stringy mane that made her feel perpetually self-conscious of her unruly mop. Bessie knew just what to do: she took Sue to her hairdresser, who chopped it down to a beautiful, short cut of naturally tight curls. Auntie Joie had dressed Sue like a waif, but Bessie bought her stylish new clothes. She

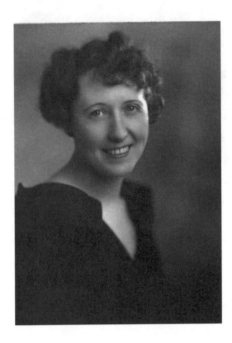

The woman who rebuilt Sue's life, her stepmother, the beloved Bessie Ross.

set out to teach the girl the "social graces" — how to serve tea, how to play mahjong, how to converse in a social setting, and how to cook. "I was her pride and joy," recalls Sue. "She turned my life around." Like Mabel File, Bessie bestowed her love unconditionally, and the effect was astonishing.

Sue attended Brandon District High School, where she joined the drama club and began to take an active role in school politics. Her marks improved, as did her popularity. With her new social skills, she became more outgoing and made friends easily.

When the war ended, Wilfrid was discharged and took a job with the Department of Veterans Affairs in Winnipeg. He purchased a home — with Bessie's money — in the upscale River Heights section of the city. Sue enrolled at Robert H.

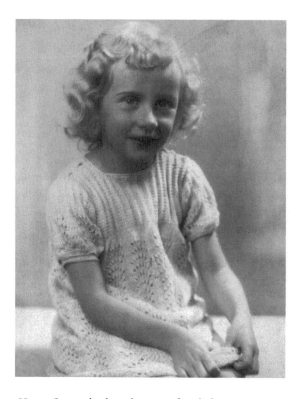

*Young Susan displays the mop of curly hair
that caused her a lifetime of consternation.*

Smith High School and then switched to Kelvin High. With her stepmother's guidance, her confidence continued to grow.

However, things weren't going well at her father's job. Wilfrid had started to drink at work. After several reprimands, he suddenly quit his job and told his wife and daughter that he could finally fulfil his ultimate dream: Wilfrid was going to build and run a summer resort. Using the last of Bessie's inheritance, he bought the charred remains of a lodge that had burned down near Kenora, Ontario. Located on Keewatin Beach Road, it was known as "Ken-O-Kee Lodge."

"He designed the absolute worst building I have ever seen," Sue shudders. "He must have been totally bombed when he designed it. It was a nightmare."

In retrospect, it was just the start of the nightmare. They lived in a small cabin on the property while the lodge was being erected by Wilfrid's drunken buddies. The cabin was not winterized. In the winter, water was shipped in by truck and stored in a cistern in the kitchen. Heating was minimal, supplied by space-heaters. Wilfrid drank heavily. He worked as a night-watchman at a garage in town, a three-mile walk since their car had died.

Bessie seemed to be drained of her usual energy. She was isolated, lonely, and ill. Sue walked to school every day, but would occasionally skip out to keep Bessie company. "When my mother was dying, I was too young to really be aware of the situation. But with Bessie, I knew something was going on. I felt so sorry for her." That winter is still a painful memory for Sue. Bessie was diagnosed with cervical cancer.

The lodge was ready by spring, and Wilfrid and his daughter actually ran it for two summers while Bessie went for treatment. The resort was a disaster. Wilfrid was soon forced to sell it at a tremendous loss, and he rented a remote cabin further from town on Lakeside Beach Road. They had no car, so Bessie's only option was to stay with friends in Lethbridge for her radiation treatments. Sue and her father were alone for the winter. "That was a terrible year, but a good year," says Sue. "It really made me strong."

Sue blasted her father for his drinking, and would pour

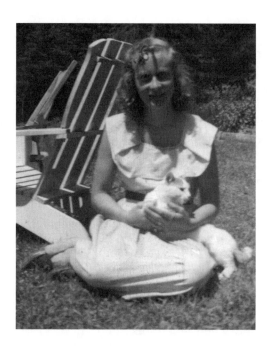

Teenaged Sue with a furry friend, probably taken at the ill-fated Ken-O-Kee Lodge.

liquor down the drain in front of him if she found any in the house. He made no protest. If he went out, she told him what time to return and threatened to lock him out in the snow if he didn't. She was fully prepared to carry out her threat, and he knew it. Drunk or not, he was always home on time. With no running water, she had to chop a hole in the ice with an axe every morning to haul water up from the lake. She chopped wood for the stove, made all the meals, did all the cleaning. She wrote to Bessie constantly. At school, she was well-liked and became president of the student council and head of the debating team. Every night, she would walk back to the cabin, miles from town, in the dark. "I don't think I had a single date in that whole time," she laughs now. "I lived too far away. No boy was ever going to walk me home!"

There was no sex on the agenda either. Her parents had never talked with her about sex, but the implicit message in her stepmother's attitude was "Don't do it!" Bessie once gave her a pamphlet published by Kotex entitled, "Now You Are A Woman." All it offered was instructions for wearing a sanitary napkin, and for personal hygiene, reinforcing the myth that female genitals have a terrible odour. That was the extent of Sue's sexual education.

"In those days, life was very different. Guys didn't expect sex. Guys didn't even try to cop a feel because they were terrified. They didn't know any more than I did, and if you got pregnant, you got married. Or you went away for a year and had the baby and put it up for adoption. You would never, ever bring the baby home. So, sex was not as much in your face."

It was also the period when her respect and affection for North American Natives took root. Sue's cabin had a phone, and Aboriginal people from the nearby reserve would often show up to use it. They would enter the cabin without knocking, offer a quiet greeting, make their call, and then thank her and leave. If she was sleeping, they would stoke the fire before they left. In the spring, she found a pair of beaded moccasins and beaded deerskin mitts on her front doorstep. She was so moved by their dignity that, to this day, she will never turn down an engagement to speak to the Aboriginal community.

By spring, Wilfrid had found employment, oddly enough, as the welfare officer for Kenora, Ontario. They rented an apartment over a store downtown and Bessie returned from out west. She had terrible radiation scars, but had survived the treatment.

During her last year of high school, Sue decided that nursing would be her career. However, the possibility of her passing chemistry was unlikely. Fate lent a hand when the school's Home Economics teacher became ill and went on sick leave. With no replacement in sight, Sue went to the principal and offered her services in exchange for receiving a perfect score in that course's exam. To her surprise, he agreed. On top of her own studies, she taught the Home Economics course during grade 13, and received a grade of 99% for it, enough to offset her poor mark in chemistry.

Although Sue was accepted for the nursing course at the Toronto General Hospital, the family could not afford to send her there. Instead, she enrolled at St. Boniface Hospital in Winnipeg. In doing so, Sue was entrusting her future to a group of women far more formidable than Auntie Joie — as Sue describes them now, the Horrible Grey Nuns.

♀♂

Joie White's fortunes had changed after Sue left Toronto.

Divorce was a rarity in those days, and Joie and her husband were still married, but legally separated. Cecil White was a powerful real estate magnate. He owned most of the Scarborough Bluffs just outside the city, an area that would become an extant, middle-class community called Rouge Hills. A main thoroughfare, White's Road, is named after him.

While in his early 40s, Cecil White suddenly dropped dead of a heart attack. His wife inherited all of his holdings, and found herself running a vast collection of properties. Joie had found her calling. She immersed herself in the business and parlayed the inheritance into an even larger fortune. Auntie

Joie had gone from being well-off to wealthy.

Sue's contact with her aunt and grandparents over the intervening years had been sporadic. They'd send the occasional letter or inexpensive Christmas gift. However, Sue's enrolment at a Catholic hospital was an affront her Protestant grandparents couldn't tolerate. Although she was their only grandchild, they disowned her from their will and never spoke to her again.

So, in the midst of her first year of training, Sue was surprised to get a phone call from her aunt. Joie informed her that her grandfather had died, and that she should come to Toronto for the funeral. Sue was too proud to say she couldn't afford to come and, to save face, lied, saying she was too busy

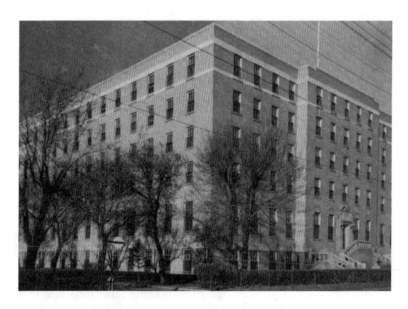

St. Boniface Teaching Hospital, Winnipeg, Manitoba, circa 1954.

with exams. She was embarrassed to ask her aunt for the plane fare, a decision she still regrets. Three days later, her grandmother died and the couple was buried in a double funeral. Joie didn't even bother to call. Sue learned of her grandmother's death over a year later.

Religious hatred was not confined to her grandparents. Sue's new masters — the Grey Nuns — felt the same about Protestants, particularly English Protestants. Susan Powell was at the top of their list.

"They were devious," says Sue, "and some of them were downright treacherous. They didn't like girls who were noncompliant. They liked Catholic girls who would behave without thinking, girls who had the makings of a future nun. They would plot against students they didn't like, almost like persecution."

The three-year nursing course was an endurance test. This was the early '50s, and students were given room and board — and $5 a month — in exchange for working shifts in the hospital as part of their training. Sue would often work a nightshift and then be expected to be in class the next morning. She recalls that, one day, she actually dozed off during a lecture and fell out of her seat onto the floor. "Leave her there!" the Sister commanded. She remained on the floor for the rest of the class. Besides exhaustion, poverty was their other great woe. The nursing students were so poor that they would take empty pop bottles from patients in the wards and cash them in. They were so hungry that they would steal food from the hospital kitchen.

One lecture that Sue stayed awake for was the one regarding birth control — one of her favourites because it was so typical of the place. She often repeats it: "The nun told us that condoms should always have holes poked in them to give sperm a fighting chance. Ha!"

In spite of her "non-compliance," Sue passed her courses, wrote her exam at the University of Manitoba, and became a registered nurse. "It was tough sledding, but I did it."

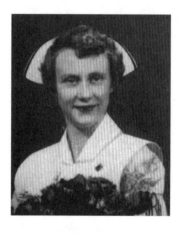

Sue's graduation photo.

While she was training, Sue would return to Kenora for visits with her parents. On one trip, an old school chum set her up on a blind date. Sue was expecting the worst, but instead she met a good-looking Swede, an electrician working for Ontario Hydro. His name was Ejnor (aye-nur) Johanson. When she returned home that night, she said to Bessie, "I've just met the man I'm going to marry." And she did, as soon as she graduated a year later.

♀♂

Sue was surprised when Auntie Joie accepted an invitation to their wedding. Joie probably came to Kenora to see what kind of fool would marry her wretched niece. To everyone's amazement, she absolutely loved Ejnor and started to keep in touch with the couple after the wedding.

Ejnor Johanson was everything Sue's father was not. He

was stalwart, dependable, responsible, and a non-drinker. Sue moved back to Kenora, happy to play the role of the quiescent spouse.

For two years, Sue worked at Kenora General Hospital, until she became pregnant and had her first daughter, Carol, in 1956. After that, Ejnor, who held very traditional views of marriage, would not allow her to work. She quickly became pregnant again. About this time, they received a mysterious invitation from Joie to come to Toronto.

It was September of 1956, and Joie White was tired of running her empire alone. She had been swindled by accountants and lawyers, and she needed someone who was thoroughly honest and dependable. She had decided that Ejnor Johanson was that person. As soon as Sue, Ejnor, and the baby arrived, Joie proposed that they move to Toronto and that Ejnor give up his job in order to work for her. During the discussion, Joie was barely civil to her niece, who was five-months pregnant at the time, and completely solicitous to Ejnor. Sue was horrified. As far as she was concerned, this was a bid for her cruel aunt to take control of her life yet again. Ejnor was appalled by Joie's treatment of his wife. He knew that accepting the offer would likely ruin his marriage. He declined and they quickly returned home. But Joie would not give up that easily.

Eric was born in 1957, and once again, Sue became pregnant right away. Unexpectedly, Ejnor received a parcel from Joie. It contained a mortgage, in the couple's name, for a new house she had built for them in one of her developments near Toronto. He sent the mortgage back, making it clear that he and Sue were happy with the path they had chosen. Their second daughter, Jane, was born in 1958, and they settled into an uneventful, suburban existence. Then, something spectacularly ironic happened.

One evening, shortly after Christmas of 1962, as Joie White sat in bed reading a book, she suffered a massive coronary attack and died. Her body was not found for three days. Sue was summoned. She hurried to Toronto to attend the funeral — and to discover an astonishing secret: Joie White had left her entire estate to Sue, her only surviving relative, on the condition that Ejnor act as executor. The estate was worth over a million dollars. In the end, Joie got her way after all.

♀♂

Suddenly, the Johansons were wealthy. They had a huge estate to manage and they could not run it from Kenora. In 1963 Ejnor quit his job, they packed up the kids, and moved to North York, a suburb of Toronto. They bought a modest home at 23 Citation Drive. In spite of their new circumstances, both Sue and Ejnor, having been raised in poverty, were addicted to frugality. To this day, Sue sews many of her own clothes and will drive miles out of her way to find the cheapest gas around.

Their new life soon took a tragic turn, however, when their fourth child, a boy, was stillborn. Sue was devastated. She salved her grief by becoming a foster parent, and, for four years, transformed their household into a refuge for a stream of babies in distress.

Sue suffered another emotional blow during this period — her beloved Bessie died. Wilfrid had purchased a derelict cabin on Longbow Lake outside of Kenora, and he and Bessie had retired there. She had been in poor health since her radical cancer treatments years earlier. Her life with Wilfrid had been one of loneliness and isolation.

"We should have bought a bigger house and had them move in with us, but we didn't," says Sue now with regret. Wilfrid was placed in Pinecrest Manor, a nursing home in Kenora, where he died four years later of hypostatic pneumonia.

"When he died, I felt a sense of relief, and a lot of guilt about leaving him up there alone. And a lot of anger at how he had treated my mom and my stepmom. Not at how he had treated me. In our relationship, I ruled. I was the strong one."

Sue's own kids were growing up, and she settled into her role as housewife and mother with a certain resignation. Like many bored homemakers, she dealt with her restlessness by taking courses in crafts like macramé and découpage. "I did everything but basket-weaving," she snickers now. A pall of predictability fell over her life.

One bright spot was her growing reputation in the neighbourhood as an adult who could talk to teens. Although her kids regarded her as completely uncool — "They called me a Neanderthal parent" — their friends were of a different opinion. The Johanson kitchen became the spot where kids would gather for lively discussions and homemade sourdough biscuits. Often the conversations would include the topic of sex.

"I was petrified to talk to my own kids about sex, but I had no problem at all talking to their friends. I never found it embarrassing or uncomfortable. Usually my kids weren't there, and I only hoped that their friends would pass the information on to them. For sure, part of my motivation was to prove to my kids that I wasn't as 'uncool' as they thought."

In 1969, her openness led to a personal crisis that defined everything that followed.

A teenage friend of her daughter's — a bright, mature girl — came to Sue privately with a problem: she was afraid she was pregnant, and didn't want her parents to know. After some consideration, Sue offered to submit a sample of the girl's urine for pregnancy testing under her own name. She did, and word soon got around Citation Drive that Sue Johanson "was knocked up again."

At that time, abortion was illegal in Canada. But that was what the girl decided she wanted. Having lost a baby herself, Sue was opposed to abortion. They discussed having the baby and putting it up for adoption. The girl could not be swayed from her decision, and, in the end, Sue realized that she had no right to make a personal choice for someone else. She drove the girl to Buffalo for the procedure.

Although the girl weathered the ordeal just fine, the traumatic event changed Sue forever. It was then and there that she found her mission — adolescents should not have to deal with unwanted pregnancies. She set out to make sure they had the personal skills and tools to prevent it.

With that fire burning, Sue went to North York City Hall and asked to see the Medical Officer of Health. This turned out to be Dr. Marguerite Archibald, a pioneer of public health in Canada. Sue stated her case plainly — she wanted to start a sexual health clinic in a high school and she wanted North York's co-operation.

At the time, Dr. Archibald was engaged in a friendly rivalry with her contemporary, Dr. Marion Powell, another pioneer of Canadian medicine. Dr. Powell had already established a public sexual health clinic in the adjoining suburb of Scarborough. Dr. Archibald saw this as an opportunity to best her. During her meeting with Sue, Dr. Archibald phoned the head of the North York Board of Education and secured a high school, Don Mills Collegiate, for the clinic.

"Okay, Mrs. Johanson, go ahead and do it," Dr. Archibald told this woman she had only just met. "But you have no budget. You'll have to get your staff and equipment on your own."

Sue set to work, finding doctors who would volunteer, cajoling nursing friends into helping out, and convincing equipment companies to donate examination tables and office furniture. Her daughters volunteered to staff the reception desk. In September 1970, Sue opened the first sexual health clinic located in a high school in North America.

"We were open one evening a week, and word quickly spread. We had kids coming from all over the city, not just North York, and even from other cities like Hamilton and Belleville. There'd be 30 to 45 students a night, lined up in the hallway, doing their homework. It was amazing."

The clinic could offer any service that didn't require parental knowledge or consent, such as birth control pills, pregnancy tests, testing for sexually transmitted diseases, and counselling. Sue ran it for the next 18 years. In order to help out with the workload, she took counselling and human sexuality courses at the University of Toronto and the Toronto Institute for Human Relations. Later, Sue attended an intensive, month-long course in Ann Arbor, Michigan, with Doctors Archibald and Powell.

"My knowledge was increasing by leaps and bounds, and I

55

started to see that these kids had absolutely no idea about sex. They needed better teaching."

Again, Sue went to her mentor, Dr. Archibald, and offered her services as a sexual education teacher. She pointed out that it was unreasonable to expect physical education instructors to teach volleyball, soccer, basketball, floor hockey, and sex.

Dr. Archibald agreed and said, "If you can get any school to invite you in, then go ahead and do it. We'll pay you the standard hourly rate."

Sue was off and running. Her first class was a Grade 9 at Cedarbrae Collegiate in Scarborough. She was so scared that when she held up a condom, she couldn't keep it from shaking violently. In spite of her nerves, the kids responded well and she loved the attention. Soon, she was being booked all over North York, then in other boroughs, and then in other cities. It snowballed rapidly — she could barely keep up.

However, Sue's new sense of self was not playing well at home. Over the years, she had transformed herself and grown; but now she felt stifled in her home life. Finally, she decided to take a year's "sabbatical" from the marriage, and rented a furnished apartment for herself. She and Ejnor entered into marriage counselling, but she couldn't deny the fact that she loved the freedom of being on her own. After a year of living alone, she moved back home briefly. When Jane, her youngest daughter, left, that was it. Sue needed independence. In 1980, she bought a condo and moved out for good.

As one might expect from Sue Johanson, this was not the typical collapse of a marriage. She and Ejnor have never divorced nor even had a legal separation, and their relationship now is probably the best it's ever been. They see each other at least twice a week, for dinner or a movie, visit at each other's cottages, and celebrate all family occasions together. They've both dated other people but there's never been any jealousy or animosity, each respecting the other's desire for some steady companionship. If there's one area they're well-matched in, it's practicality. Ejnor continues to manage the original estate, which has prospered over the years. "I trust Ejnor absolutely, one hundred percent," says Sue. "I just don't want to live with him. In fact, I don't want to live with anybody."

Meanwhile, her reputation as someone who could talk to kids about sex continued to grow. In the evenings, she would take more courses or teach parents how to talk to their own children about sexuality. Sue believes that sexual education is a parent's responsibility, but she knows from personal experience how tough that can be.

Sue's love affair with the media began in 1984 when the Toronto *Sun* printed a full-page article about an ebullient sexual educator working in North York schools. Suddenly, Sue was getting calls from *Canada AM* and CBC. Journalist Jane Hawtin invited her on to her radio show, *Barometer*, at Q107. After the interview, Jane said cryptically, "Stop by and see the station manager on the way out, will you Sue? He wants to talk to you."

The station manager was the mercurial Gary Slaight, whose family owned the station and many others. He was sitting in his office, leaning back in his chair with his feet, clad in red running shoes, propped up on the desk.

"Sue, how would you like to do a weekly phone-in show for kids about sex?" he asked. She jumped at the chance. "Fine. I'll pay you $25 for a two-hour show and you start this Sunday night." It was Thursday.

Sue left in a panic, rushing home to ponder what she had gotten herself into. Then, accepting her fate, she started rounding up research — enough to fill an entire program if no one called in. The opposite proved to be the case: the lines were jammed right from the start. Since there was initially no call-screener, the engineer would go through the questions while Sue was talking on air. They would then play some music while Sue picked out which call she wanted next.

"There I was, sandwiched between Van Halen and Guns N' Roses," she laughs.

She got into trouble on the very first night:

"A question came through about bum sex, although I think he said, 'Sex in the asshole.' Well, I wasn't going to say that. I was trying to explain the dangers of anal sex, and I was trying to think of a word to say instead of 'shit.' I couldn't say 'faeces' because this audience was not going to know that, or 'defecation,' so I said 'caca.' Well, Allan Slaight, Gary's dad, was listening and he called Gary the next day, complaining bitterly about this woman on his station saying 'caca.' So, I got called in and simply said to Gary, 'Okay, what do you want me to call it? Poo-poo? Doo-doo? Crap? Number 2? Shit?' And finally, I said 'caca.' 'Caca' is one that everybody understands, it's not offensive, and you know what I'm talking about. And he had to agree."

Eventually, the show started airing coast to coast on the Rock Radio Network. Sue did 50 shows a year for the next 14 years. After a fight with Gary, she also got a raise after the third season — to $75 a week.

"I loved doing radio. I realized that I am very good with words, and that the brain really works well — you know, you can't always rely on the brain at other times — but when I'm on radio or television, that brain is working. It's working hard. It makes me feel alive and in control. And," she adds, " I have to be honest — it's an ego trip."

After doing Q107 for a year, Sue approached Rogers Cable in Toronto about doing a weekly television show entitled "Talk Sex." Again, it was a phone-in show aimed at young people. Producer Don Adams liked the idea, and the show went into production in 1985. Every Thursday night for 11 years, Sue Johanson was available for advice on the local community access channel for all of Rogers's subscribers. Most of that time, she worked for free.

In 1996, WTN fulfilled Sue's dream of hosting a national, phone-in, television show, the *Sunday Night Sex Show*. She's well-paid now, but that's not the point, and neither is the ego massage.

"Dr. Archibald once said to me, 'None of us does one damn thing that doesn't meet our needs,' and I never forgot that," she says. Sue's need is to prove to Auntie Joie that she's not the loser Joie believed her to be; to take her revenge on the cruel Grey Nuns; to prove to her family that she's not the mousy, suburban mother they grew up with; and to prove to the world that Wilfrid's daughter has the strength of character he lost along the way. Her mission is her proof, and she lives by it — or will, at the very least, go down fighting.

♀♂

It's December of 2000. I'm sitting in my former office at CTV when the phone rings.

"Guess what?" It's Sue, and she's really excited.

"What?"

"I just got the Order of Canada!" She starts to cry.

"Congratulations! I hate to tell you this, but I know already."

Indeed, I did. Receiving the Order of Canada is a long, bureaucratic process. Eight months earlier, the Governor-General's office had contacted WTN, looking for information about Sue's birthplace and date. In turn, Julie had contacted me,

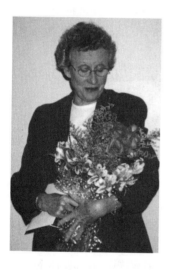

When Sue's Order of Canada was announced, the crew presented her with a gorgeous bouquet.

and we were all sworn to secrecy with the threat of having to scrub floors in Rideau Hall. I confessed my secret involvement to Sue.

"You know, it came in this big envelope with a government logo on it," she says, "and when I saw it, I just thought, 'I can't believe they want their fucking GST already!' And then I opened it, and it's from the Governor General! I can't believe it!" More tears. "Oh, if Joie could see me now."

The Order of Canada is the Canadian equivalent of being knighted. Any Canadian citizen can be nominated. Worthy nominees are presented the award by the Governor-General, the Queen's representative. Although Sue holds the Royal Family in low regard, her British ancestry got the better of her in this instance, and she was completely overwhelmed. No award could have meant more to her. It was public recognition for a lifetime of public service.

When that public service will end is anybody's guess. Sue has no intention of retiring, although she has slowed down. She stopped the radio show in 1998, mainly because it was cutting into her summers too much. From May until September, she stays at her cottage on Lake Simcoe, and driving back and forth to Toronto every Sunday night was taking its toll. She continues to do public speaking engagements, usually at universities and colleges, but she has cut that back to 50 speaks a year. The *Sunday Night Sex Show* requires 30 appearances a season, which ends in May. In addition, Sue continues to write regular newspaper columns and does television interviews on various sexual topics. She may have cut back, but she's not exactly slacking off.

Her cottage is her refuge and it keeps her forever busy — tending gardens, making preserves, cleaning spiders off the boathouse, painting and repainting. Every morning, she walks five kilometres with Peggy, her friend from across the road, and rides her bike twice that distance after supper every night. She bakes, she sews, she swims, she visits with her husband, children, and grandchildren. All summer long, she's out at yard sales every Saturday morning, arguing down prices with exasperated homeowners. (She's so cheap, she'll fight to have a 10-cent item reduced to a nickel.) In short, she maintains a pace that would kill a 35-year-old.

Some people are blessed with an abundance of energy, and Sue is such a person. I think the secret is that she sleeps so well. I've seen her sleep through a tornado and then wake up the next morning wondering why there's a tree missing out back.

The winters she spends at her condo in Toronto. Of course, she's the vice-president of her condominium building. Most weeks, she's on the road doing lectures, anywhere from Yellowknife to St. John's. At one point, she had accumulated 200,000 air miles. All she wanted to do was go to her cottage.

However, the Order of Canada made Sue throw her frugality out the window. For the presentation, she booked a *first class* train ticket (at the government's expense, of course) to Ottawa and took her eldest daughter, Carol, along for company. Of course, Sue saved money by buying her formal dress at a store-closing sale for $29. Regardless, she looked elegant in black, with a string of pearls around her neck, as she marched up the aisle on May 31, 2001 to accept her award from Governor-General Adrienne Clarkson.

Up to that point, the proceedings had been predictably staid, orderly, and dull. As might be expected, Sue's arrival took care of that.

Although Sue was on her best behaviour, the poor announcer suffered a slip of the tongue as she introduced the illustrious guest:

"Miss Sue Johanson. She's been a strong sexual advocate. . . ."

The announcer abruptly stopped, shocked at what she had said. Sue, the Governor-General, and the entire cadre of distinguished recipients looked stunned, then burst out laughing.

"Forgive me," the announcer implored Sue as the laughter swelled. "I'm sorry."

Sue just gave her two thumbs up and roared. As the mirth subsided, the announcer began again without a stumble:

"She has been a strong, successful advocate for sex education in Canada over the last three decades. She's known for her nationally televised *Sunday Night Sex Show* and for her Toronto-based radio call-in show. She is a popular figure with adolescents and young adults. A registered nurse, she opened one of the city's first birth control clinics and has talked to thousands of students in high schools, colleges and universities across the country. Candid in her responses, she helps Canadians to understand their sexuality and health choices. Miss Sue Johanson."

As Sue beamed with pride, Governor-General Clarkson, a former broadcaster herself, pinned the Order of Canada over Sue's heart. To all of us who know her well, that could have been anywhere on her body.

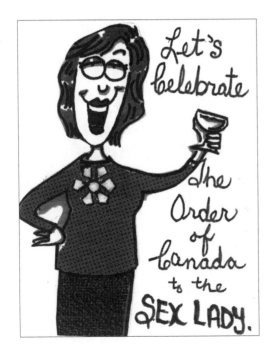

Sue's homemade invitation.

From Kenora to Kansas

In January 2002, a most curious thing happened.

The American cable channel, Oxygen, purchased 26 taped episodes of the *Sunday Night Sex Show*. Timorously, they began airing the show two nights a week at 1:00 a.m. Not exactly a stellar time-slot, but — just like WTN seven years earlier — they were afraid of a potential public backlash.

After seven years, Canadians are comfortable with Sue's frankness, but turning her loose on American audiences, complete with her exuberant explanations of blow-jobs and bum sex, was a dicey proposition. Oxygen execs clutched their desks, white-knuckled, waiting to be swept overboard by a tidal wave of subscriber cancellations.

In fact, just the opposite happened. There was a flood of calls raving about this "new" show. By March, Oxygen Media had bought the U.S. rights to the entire seven seasons of the *Sunday Night Sex Show*. It is now one of their highest rated shows.

Because these were taped shows, American viewers were frustrated that they couldn't phone in. Oxygen asked Sue about doing a live program specifically for the United States. Sue's initial reluctance disappeared when she met the folks at Oxygen in New York; she couldn't resist their warmth, humour, and sincerity.

So, *Talk Sex with Sue Johanson* began airing weekly on November 3, 2002. Sue has set up a Web site with answers to the most commonly asked questions at www.talksexwithsue.com.

After a lifetime of setting trends, Sue had done it again. *Talk Sex* became the first, live phone-in show ever to be sold from Canada to the U.S. Not bad for a nurse from Kenora.

Live

"Two minutes to air," Liisa announces.

Everyone has been on headsets for several minutes now, reviewing their tasks and checking their equipment. Sue is deep in thought on the set, focusing on the broadcast. Liz, Liisa, and I are positioned at the front desk in the Control Room, and Dwayne is beside us in the glassed-in audio booth. There's a wall of monitors in front of us. Sana and Sheldon, the technical producer, are sitting behind us. At the rear of the room, Mona has been lining up calls for the last half-hour — six callers are on hold, waiting for their chance to talk to Sue.

"Two minutes," I say to Sue in her IFB (Interrupted Fold Back) earpiece.

"Two minutes," she announces to the studio crew, although they had heard both Liisa and I.

The headsets feed the audio output of the show to everyone, as well as my mic and Liisa's mic. As I discovered years ago, it's not a good idea to eat potato chips while every-

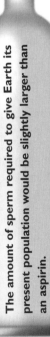

The amount of sperm required to give Earth its present population would be slightly larger than an aspirin.

one is on headset. They get really peeved at the sound of amplified crunching. In addition, each person has an intercom key at their post, and can address individual headsets or all of them if the need arises ("Stop crunching!").

"Okay, Liisa and Ali, here's the first two callers." It's Julie from the call-screening booth. "Joan, from Halifax. Joan from Halifax. That's the first caller. And Michael, from Edmonton. Michael from Edmonton. That's the second caller. Did you get those?"

"Yes Julie," Ali responds from the studio.

Liisa says, "Yup. Minute and a half to air." I've written the names on my rundown, and she's quickly typing both names into the character generator. A character generator, which sounds like something from _The Matrix_, is the gizmo that

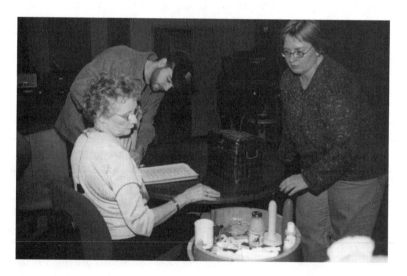

Derrick mics Sue for rehearsal, while Frances checks the standard props on the side table.

displays names on air. Typed text is commonly referred to as "supers," as in "superimposed." Out of the corner of my eye, I notice on the prompter monitor that Ali is also typing in the names and locations. Germain wanders into the shot behind Sue, and moves her wooden dollies to a better position. Sue is looking a tad tired and I open my key to Harvey in video:

"Harvey, can you soften the cameras a wee bit?" Both images lose some detail.

"How's that?" he asks.

"Good. Thanks." Softening a shot is a wonderful antidote to ageing, as Angela Lansbury ably demonstrated weekly on *Murder She Wrote*.

"One minute to air." Liisa is counting to 22:59:55 Eastern time, the actual time we start the show. Because of a five-second delay, we start five seconds before 11:00 p.m. She's following the master clock in the Control Room, which she had synchronized with Master Control in Winnipeg earlier in the evening.

"One minute," I tell Sue. She nods on the monitor, looking down at her notes. "We'll be coming to camera 2."

"Camera 2," she repeats, glancing up and smiling at Derrick behind the camera. He adjusts his framing to match her headroom.

Sue is hard of hearing, and, although she owns a hearing-aid, she rarely wears it. She finds its amplified crush of noise intolerable, not unlike potato chips crunching, I suppose. For this situation, the IFB functions as her hearing-aid, since Dwayne can control the level of audio going into it. Sue hears herself at 80% and the caller at 100%. Either Dwayne or I can speak to her, and, if we do, the caller's level drops during the time we have our intercom keys open. I've learned to use this function sparingly since she has a habit of repeating whatever it is I say to her. "Sue, hold the book up." Sue, on air, says, "I loved this book, hold the book up, by Dr. Yosh Taguchi."

"Can you ask Sue to straighten her collar?" Sana asks. She has a keen eye for dishevelment.

"Derrick, can you straighten Sue's collar please?" I ask. We have all been conditioned to preen ourselves in front of a mirror, and it's difficult to tidy your own appearance while watching a monitor. When your image is not reversed, movement seems entirely unnatural. We see his camera jiggle as he locks it off, and then he's in the shot, gently primping the top of her jacket.

"Thirty seconds to air."

"Thirty seconds, Sue," I tell her.

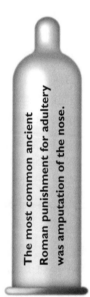

The most common ancient Roman punishment for adultery was amputation of the nose.

"Thirty seconds," she says to Derrick, who is still fussing with her. "Good old Susie," she smiles at him. "Always looking like a tramp."

"We just can't take you anywhere," I say in her IFB. She chuckles as Derrick leaves the set.

"Only to bingo," she laughs.

"Happy, Sana?" I turn to her.

"That's better."

I open my key to videotape. "Stand by the opening, Ivan."

"Standing by," he answers.

"Fifteen seconds." Liisa checks her stopwatch.

It's time for the ritual benediction. When Adrian Hepes worked on the show as the technical producer, he would address all of us via intercom at this point, and say, with his Romanian accent, "Have a good show everybody." Before he left, he kindly left his declaration on an audio cart for us, and Dwayne plays it on cue:

"Half a gude show every bawdy."

We answer as a chorus. "Thanks Adrian."

Liisa starts her countdown. "Ten seconds, nine, eight, seven, six . . ."

"Five to opening, Sue," I tell her.

"Four, three, two . . ."

"Roll tape." I see on the tape playback monitor that Ivan has rolled it.

"One."

"Up on it," I say to Liz. She brings up the fader on the switcher, and the *Sunday Night Sex Show* animation and music flow on a stream of electrons from Toronto to Winnipeg. I glance up at the off-air monitor, which is tuned to WTN, and see the show start there five seconds later.

"Twenty seconds to studio."

Sue is listening to the opening music and bopping in her seat, revving up her own energy level for the upcoming hour.

"Coming to you, Sue. Camera 2. Better watch out — Sheldon just saw the 'Squirmy Vagina' in the hallway."

She laughs.

"Ten to studio, nine, eight, seven . . ."

I echo Liisa's count on Sue's IFB, "Six to you, five, four, three, coming to camera two, one. Dissolve."

Liz dissolves from tape to Derrick's camera. He slowly zooms in, as always.

"You're up!" I say to Sue.

She starts, full of life. "I'm Sue Johanson and we have another exciting *Sunday Night Sex Show* for you this week."

Too late to turn back now.

♀♂

The word "live" is a word that can strike terror into the hearts of many a seasoned television pro.

Being involved in a live broadcast is living on the edge, the television equivalent of walking over the Niagara Gorge on a tightrope or accepting a ride home from Chuck Yeagher.

There are so many things that can go wrong: technical elements can go awry, the transmission can cut out, lights can burn out, cameras can die, microphones can fail, wrong shots can be taken, wrong tapes can roll, tapes can jam, name supers can be spelled wrong, the host can cough or sneeze — or worse, freeze up. Compound all those variables with the addition of live phone calls from viewers, and you've got a mix that's as stable as Ross Perot on a bobsled.

Then there are those of us who love it. All those things that can go wrong do, and dodging them is more fun than a paintball shoot-out. In this business, nothing matches the exhilaration of confronting a live broadcast and conquering it. Viewers sense the jangled nerves behind the scenes. On air, it translates into a pulse of energy, adding an aura of unpredictability to a show that is far more real than the "reality" of an edited program such as *Survivor*. Best of all, a live show starts on time and ends on time. No dawdling for hours trying to tweak a shot or insert a graphic. What you see is what you get. Period.

Visiting the Control Room during a show leaves most folks

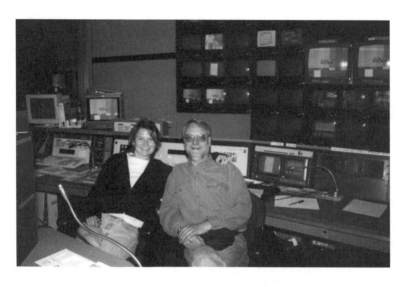

Stacey White, our other favourite Technical Director, and RJ in the Control Room. It's 15 minutes to air, and you can see how tense we are.

completely baffled, as if they're in Mission Control at a NASA launch, trying to figure out what the hell all those people are doing. Although viewers only see Sue, and occasionally Germain, on air they're aware that there's a staff working behind the scenes. What surprises viewers is that it takes 17 people to put that simple show format of one person answering phone calls on the screen. Here's the team involved:

1. Host
2. Producer — controls the content of the show; meddles with the direction.
3. Director — controls the look of the show; meddles with the content.
4. Technical producer — oversees complete technical

set-up, including satellite transmission and crew.

5. Technical director — switches cameras and oversees studio technical set up.
6. Lighting director — designs and maintains lighting.
7. Audio — mics, music, and mixing.
8. Assistant director — timing, adding name supers, and coordinating broadcast with Master Control in Winnipeg.
9. Cameraman.
10. Cameraman.
11. Teleprompter operator.
12. Call screener.
13. Video operator — controls the camera video levels throughout the show.
14. Make-up.
15. Videotape operator — plays back taped items and records the show.
16. Engineer — on stand-by for technical problems.
17. Sue's assistant — sets up Sue's props and brings water or whatever in breaks.

There's a traditional position we've never filled — floor director. Normally, this person counts the host in and out of segments and assists in the studio. On the *Sunday Night Sex Show*, I count Sue in and out through her IFB ear-piece. Derrick and Germain help her out on the floor. Also, there's an additional job that is peculiar to SkyDome alone — the "beer-barrel guard."

Early in our tenure at Dome Productions, there were a couple of shows where we could hear thunder in the background. Viewers across the country must have thought, "My, they have a lot of storms in Toronto." We'd leave the studio with our umbrellas at the ready, but the pavement outside would be perfectly dry. We'd think, "My, what a short storm." After two weeks of unnaturally brief thunderstorms, the real source of the rumbling was uncovered. Above the studio is a supply area, and workers were rolling dollies loaded with beer cases in and out of the stadium after events. It sounded exactly like beer-barrels being rolled and we expected Walter Ostanek to strike up the accordion at any moment. The problem was solved by placing a "beer-barrel guard," usually a student, in that area when required. They are quite prepared to throw themselves under a dolly or slap Walter silly, if necessary.

During the show, there are actually six separate areas that work together:

1. The Studio — Host, two cameramen, teleprompter operator, and lighting director.

2. Control Room — Technical director, technical producer, director, audio person, assistant director and make-up.

3. Call-screening area — Producer, call screener, and Sue's assistant. This area is a glassed-in booth at the rear of the Control Room.

4. Video — Video operator, controlling camera levels and quality. Located down the hall from the Control Room.

5. Videotape — Tape operator. Located one floor below the studio area.

6. WTN Master Control — Located in Winnipeg. All programs air through Master, where commercials are inserted.

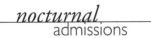
The program is transmitted to Winnipeg, where a five-second delay is added, and then re-broadcast by satellite coast to coast. This complicated mix is coordinated, in theory, by the director, although the assistant director deals with Master Control via intercom. People ask me how one can keep track of all those elements and I always tell them that directing is like doing air traffic control except nobody gets killed.

The five-second delay exists for one purpose — in case someone says something naughty on air. If that happens, the delay allows Winnipeg time to cut the audio. Oddly, considering the nature of the program, it never has.

An orgasm lasts approximately 3 to 10 seconds.

"I was a bit frightened at first that there'd be foul language," admits producer Julie Smith. "I had no idea of the respect that viewers and listeners had for Sue. I'd listened to Sue's show on the radio myself years before, and it became clear, quite quickly, that people struggled for the right terminology because of respect for her. Sure, there's a couple of idiots here and there, but the average person who phones in has a love and respect for Sue, and will try to use the right terms."

The fact that there are viewers at all is attributable to the leap of faith made by one woman in Winnipeg.

♀♂

In September 1995, Susan Millican, the vice-president of programming for the fledgling Women's Television Network, WTN, was sitting in her office watching the network's morning

74

show, *Call Us*. The live program, broadcast from the company's headquarters in Winnipeg, was featuring a phone-in segment with guest Sue Johanson.

Millican was aware of the sexual educator, and had, in fact, attended one of her lectures while still in university. Susan had enjoyed Sue's presentation at the time, but it had never occurred to her that Sue's explicit frankness would be acceptable on television. Watching her that morning, she started to think differently.

Suddenly, the vice-president of engineering, Carol Darling, burst into her office. "Are you watching this woman?" she asked excitedly. "She's amazing!"

They watched the rest of the segment together and decided, on the spur of the moment, to offer Sue her own show on WTN.

"I was struck by her courage and her candour," Susan recalls. "She was such a great example of a strong woman, a positive image we were trying to convey. Plus, it was the beginning of our license and we needed some ratings."

Susan and Carol invited Sue to lunch after the broadcast and they headed off to Earl's, a trendy eatery in the Polo Park district of Winnipeg. The three of them hit it off immediately and Susan was impressed by Sue's sincerity. "She's so honest and caring about people. She clearly was not doing this for self-aggrandizement." During the course of the meal, Susan suggested a weekly national show to be broadcast from Winnipeg, which would've required Sue to commute from Toronto every Sunday. Sue listened politely, but commented to me when she returned, "They're crazy if they think I'm going to fly out to Winnipeg every weekend." She was enthusiastic about the show and WTN; but the commute was going to be the deal-breaker. Susan Millican was not going to let that happen.

Susan knew in her gut that the time was right for the show, even though her two sons, who were both attending a private Jesuit school, told her she was "out of her mind." She was raised Catholic, the type of figure that Sue's grandfather, James Bell, would have railed against. Yet she sensed that the timing was right for a national broadcast of Sue Johanson's mission. She proposed renting a studio in Toronto and broadcasting from there. Sue accepted the offer with glee.

Susan Millican says, "If we'd just wanted the ratings, we would have hired some blonde bimbo. Sue Johanson is *the* pioneer of sexual education in Canada. She's frank without being sensational, and she's totally trustworthy. The fact that she looks like a grandmother just adds to her appeal."

Initially, the program was entitled, "Sex With Sue."

"The problem was that I'd be phoning around for sponsors," Susan Millican laughs, "and I'd have to leave a message that said I was calling with regards to 'Sex With Sue.' Well, it was getting a little embarrassing and I knew we had to change *that!*"

She also knew there'd be complaints about the nature of the show, but she trusted Sue. "The show is not about titillation. It's educational and informational and that falls within the broadcast standards guidelines."

Susan's respect for Sue is returned in kind. They share a natural, unpretentious warmth and a personal commitment to public service. Susan Millican was one of the select few invited to Sue's private, Order of Canada celebration. She made the journey all the way from Winnipeg just for the afternoon. "Her lectures alone, even without radio and television, have

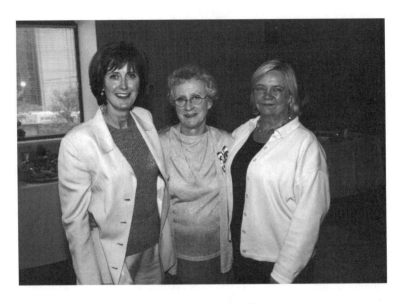

Susan Millican, Sue, and Julie Smith at Sue's Order of Canada brunch.

helped thousands of Canadians to have better lives," Susan says. "She really deserved it."

It fell to Julie Smith, the head of independent production, to organize the *Sunday Night Sex Show*.

"Susan contacted me and said, 'We're going to do the show as an in-house, studio-based production and we need a producer.' And I said, 'Well, jeepers, I'd love to produce it because I've never done live TV before.' So my original intention was to work only on the first 13 episodes — you know, setting up the studio, getting the crew together, overseeing it a bit, and then handing it over — but I got so hooked on the adrenaline and the people that there was no way on earth I was giving it up!"

♀♂

"Did we beat Julie?"

The three of us — Sue, Frances, and I — invariably ask each other this question as we pull into the parking lot before the show.

Sue and I usually have supper together at my place on Sunday evening before going to work. If she arrives early, she sits out front of my house in her car, listening to Rex Murphy on CBC Radio. "I have to admit I have the hots for Rex Murphy," she says. Her other great heartthrob is General Lewis McKenzie, whom she finds irresistibly sexy. We take turns cooking, and I definitely get the better of that deal. Sue will make Swedish meatballs with fresh beets and an asparagus salad; I'll do hot dogs and Fritos.

Frances meets us as we're loading the car with our essential gear — Sue's tote bag containing her sex toys and books, her wardrobe, a batch of sourdough biscuits, and my collapsible Z-Scooter. I won the scooter at Jumbo Video two years ago, and it's become an invaluable television tool. With the layout at SkyDome, the studio is so far from the Control Room that Dwayne and I are forever zipping up and down the narrow hall like a couple of overgrown schoolboys on the tear.

"There's her car," Frances says, spotting it first. We never arrive before Julie, and if we did, we'd probably panic and drive around in circles until she got there.

As we unload the car, Liisa pulls up beside us, bright and pert as always.

"Hi everyone. How was your week?" she asks, giving Sue a hug.

"Oh, it was great! I was out in the Maritimes, doing speaks in Halifax and Fredericton," Sue responds. "How 'bout you? Busy this week?"

The kibitzing starts in the parking lot and continues from there. It's Sunday evening, time for the regular family visit. It certainly doesn't feel like we're going to work, but we are. Julie is amiably yapping away with Priya in the boardroom when we arrive.

The workday begins at 8:00 p.m. with the production meeting. We go over the night's script, check Sue's research, and discuss upcoming episodes and toys. By its nature, most of the show is unscripted, but Sue writes some sections ahead of time —

> Masters and Johnson reported that 3 males per 1000 perform self-fellatio.

her opening and closing; the "Pleasure Chest"; "FYI Sex," which is medical information relating to sexual health; and a book review. Sometimes these are written months before they air, often in the summer while she's at the cottage.

Most programs suffer from a hierarchy where the production staff and the crew are divided into two camps that have little to do with each other. Those in production tend to think of technical staff as coddled, whiny, manual labourers who are devoid of creative impulse; the crew regard production people with disdain, as third-rate talents who exhibit neither technical competence nor realistic expectations. Part of the director's job is to act as a buffer between the two factions. However, these prevailing attitudes could not be further from the reality of the *Sunday Night Sex Show.*

During the production meeting, we leave the double doors of the boardroom wide open. Everyone arriving has to walk by those doors, and everyone waves or stops in to say "Hi." Lynda Debono, who was our original call-screener, points out: "Just the fact that you have the doors open — it's the sense that people can walk in freely and say hello. That's a really neat thing. I've never seen that on any other production."

While we have our meeting, the studio guys set up their cameras and help with the lights. In the Control Room, Liisa types in the "bumpers" — "Sue's Quickies" and resource pages — while Liz lines up videotapes with Ivan. Dwayne sets up audio and tests the phone lines, usually with Germain's help. Like a well-rehearsed military manoeuvre, all the pieces and people fall into place. But it was not always thus.

♀♂

"Try to book crew members who are open-minded," Julie said to Chris Priess, the technical producer. It was December 1995, and we were in our first pre-production meeting for the new WTN program, the *Sunday Night Sex Show*. It was the first time I'd met Julie — who was looking very officious, bristling in a business suit — and Chris, whom I knew only by reputation. He had worked on a show some of my colleagues had endured, the maudlin *Shirley* show, for CTV. Julie had chosen the same facility, Electric Images, for Sue's first national television effort, and I was apprehensive. The fact that Chris turned bright red each time Julie mentioned the word "sex" did not soothe my nerves.

"Plus, we're going to need some electronic graphics done

for the monitor behind Sue," Julie added, pulling a brochure out of her briefcase. "These are medical drawings of reproductive systems, male and female, that Sue can use for reference." The very shy Chris looked at the illustrations — female genitals, frontal; non-erect penis; erect penis; erect penis with condom — and turned into a tomato. His embarrassment was soon avenged.

"When we were first starting the show," Julie admits, "I was in my straight-backed producer mode, didn't have a clue what I was doing. Naturally, when you don't have a clue what you're doing, you're more petrified than normal. So, sure enough, they called me a week later and said the graphics were ready. So, I trot over there with my producer hat on, all official, and I walk into this control room, and on every single monitor in the room — which was a number of monitors — they had this spread-eagled female genitalia. You can imagine walking into a room full of pussy. Well, these guys are all looking at me, waiting for me to crumble. I thought, 'Oh my God, I want to die,' but I couldn't die with all these men looking at me. So, I looked at it and, in my efficient producer voice said, 'Yes, everything seems to be in the right place. Next.'"

Her only other comment was that, on the graphic of the erect penis, the testicles looked too big. Every man in the room uncrossed his legs.

Chris, a baby-faced, thirty-something guy with considerable technical acumen, worked on the show for several years. He believes that Julie's choice of a small facility to produce the program was a clever decision.

"The fact that Electric Images was a small company made the show more like a small-town production. If she had gone to a big studio, like CBC, the *Sunday Night Sex Show* wouldn't have had the same consistency of crew every week, and that would have totally changed the flavour of the show."

Since the first 13 episodes were only a trial, the budget for the program was minuscule. The set — which had deep-purple, free-standing flats and a small, round desk — was designed by Sean Breaugh and cost a grand total of $3,200 — less than a used car. Of course, Sue would have knitted the set for free if that had been possible.

The most complicated aspect of the production was the radio show. For the first three seasons, Sue continued to do her radio program for the first hour, and then simulcast radio and television for the second. This meant that, starting an hour before our television time-slot, Sue, the audio person, and the call-screener were tied up with radio. Sue would actually do this in an audio booth on another floor, and then race to the television studio in a commercial break with her mic cords dangling and her IFB flopping out of her ear.

For three years, the supervision of this mad dash fell to Shanda Deziel, who is now a section editor at *Maclean's* magazine. When she joined the show in its second season as Sue's assistant, the 23-year-old Shanda had a Master's degree in English and was working at Nevada Bob's Golf Shop. A tiny person with a charismatic intelligence, I was so impressed by Shanda after meeting her at a party that, when the job of Sue's assistant came up, we offered it to her. Unlike the rest of the crew, she had never heard of Sue: "I had never seen her at school so I didn't know anything about her, but when I started telling people I was going to do this, of course, everyone was like, 'Oh Sue!' *They* had lots to tell me about it."

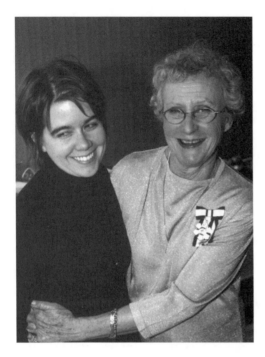

*Shanda Deziel and
Sue snuggle up at the
Order of Canada
brunch.*

(Just a note on the merits of parties: the day after we offered Shanda this minor position, someone else who was at the same party offered her a research job at *Maclean's*. She accepted both offers, and Nevada Bob's was the poorer for it. How come they never show *that* in beer commercials?)

Shanda quickly realized that, considering the random nature of viewers' calls, the rest of Sue's presentation had to be thoroughly structured. If Sue was answering a question about female condoms, for example, she didn't have time to go rooting through a box looking for one in the middle of a live show. After conferring with the host, Shanda set up all the props on a side-table in a concise order, an order that she followed religiously week after week. If Sue had to reach for something in a hurry, it was always in the same spot. "I'd obsess over where I placed everything," Shanda chuckles.

"I also got to test all those vibrators before the show, to make sure the batteries were working. It was sort of this guilty pleasure. I'd never seen one before I worked on the show; I had no idea about any of these sex toys, so it's like I had my own little, special time with dildos and vibrators. It was great!"

The wooden dolls, which Sue painted herself, were more of a problem for Shanda.

"I don't know how many times a foot or an arm fell off seconds before the show started. I was forever walking around with a foot in my pocket."

Shanda often found herself futzing with props in the studio alone with Ali, who was working at his keyboard on the script. Being a writer himself, he took an avid interest in her work at *Maclean's*, where she was struggling to establish herself. "He wanted to read almost every word I wrote," she says, "and was always so encouraging and supportive. His support meant a lot to me and that was one of the great things about being on that show."

One of the assistant's most crucial tasks is rounding up treats for the crew. Often, this means cookies, and Shanda would find herself trudging through snow on a Sunday afternoon to Kensington Market or Second Cup, hunting for the most extravagant cookies she could find. As much as she hated rounding them up, she found an odd domestic comfort in presenting them:

"I loved the cookies. I loved setting them up on the plate. I wouldn't just lay them out — I'd have to walk to each person and give them their cookies. The Control Room was always really happy and I'd set out a separate plate for the studio. I'd walk down to Sana's room and give one to Sana. I'd offer one to Sue, but Sue never ate the cookies. But, if I had Turtles, she'd eat the Turtles. I'd walk into the studio and I'd just light up. Here are these three guys — Derrick, Germain, and Ali — who are all amazing and handsome. They were just so happy and so interested and so playful with Sue. It felt like walking in with three brothers. I'd go in there with a plate of cookies, three for each of them, and every week they knew I was going to do it and they were just as excited as the week before." She reflects a moment, and then adds with an embarrassed grin, "I was so weird about the cookies that I was jealous if Sue brought in baking, because they were supposed to eat *my* cookies!"

♀♂

In the end, it fell to Lynda Debono to book the crew for the *Sunday Night Sex Show*. Her older brother, David, owned Electric Images and she'd been working there for three years as a studio manager. Her background was in the performing arts, but she had supported herself in university with a part-time job as a debt collector for the Bank of Nova Scotia. The telephone skills from that thankless experience turned out to be a major asset for the show.

"I was in an internal meeting with Chris Priess, and my brothers David and Terry," recalls Lynda, "and we were talking about the logistics for doing the show and the crew we were going to need. Chris said, 'We're going to need a call screener and I don't know who we're going to get.' I don't have a background in sex — I hadn't even had sex in a while," she laughs, "and I just said, 'I want to do that and I don't want to get paid for it.' Chris looked at me with that beet-red face and that sort of serious look like he was about to tell me off, and said, 'You can't do it. This has to be serious. You're going to giggle!' From that moment, it was almost like a challenge, and I said, 'I'm up for it.'"

Initially, she thought the show would receive mostly "obscene calls from dirty old men." Sue primed Lynda for the job by supplying her own three books to read. It was a memorable meeting:

"I remember Sue coming in and setting her bag on my desk. She had a quilted tote bag she'd made to keep her props in. She was chatting away, and I was still a little bit intimidated, and I kept hearing this noise. I didn't know what it was but I didn't even hear a word Sue said. I just kept thinking, 'What's going on?' and then I looked down at the bag, and it's moving across my desk! A vibrator had switched on and was vibrating away. I laughed so hard and thought, 'This is a great opportunity.'"

Apparently it was. Lynda is now Vice President, Post and Studio Production Services for Alliance Atlantis Broadcasting.

It was Lynda and Julie who invented "Mona Long."

Mona Long is the pseudonym of whoever the call-screener is for that episode. It could be one of several women who rotate through the position, but because the calls, by nature, are so intimate, we decided early on to keep the identity of the call-screener private. Many callers also use a false name, and, if they are from a small town, we encourage them to pick their closest urban centre as their location. Even though they are in

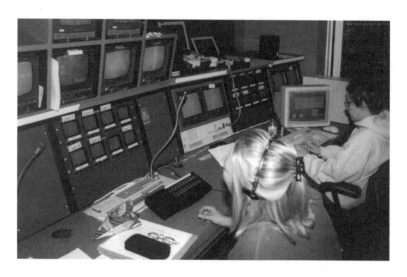

The Call Screening Room: Julie monitors the program while Shanda Deziel plays "Mona Long."

a public forum, we try to allow people as much privacy as possible under the circumstances.

From her experience as a phonecentre debt collector, Lynda had developed keen instincts for spotting bullshit. She displayed an uncanny ability to weed out the legitimate calls from the prank-calls right from the start. By her estimation, about 20% of the calls we receive are pranks, often from a student dorm or frat-house. Lynda also developed the line of patter that greets each caller:

"*Sunday Night Sex Show*. Can I get your name please?"

"Willy."

"Willy, where are you calling from?"

"Lethbridge."

"What's your question for Sue?"

During the first season, Lynda got a bit cocky about her screening abilities, so Derrick decided to send her up. About 10 minutes before a show, he went into the reception area of Electric Images and phoned our 800 number. Lynda answered:

"*Sunday Night Sex Show.* Can I get your name please?"

"Bob."

"Bob, where are you calling from?"

"B.C."

"What's your question for Sue?"

"I've got this growth coming out of the side of my penis."

"Have you talked with your doctor about this?"

"No, not yet."

"How big is it?"

"Well, it started off small but now it's about two inches long. Could it be a second penis growing?"

"I don't know, Bob. I'm going to put you on hold."

At this point, she leapt up from the phone console and ran to the front of the Control Room.

"Guys, you're not going to believe this. There's a guy on the phone who says he's growing a second penis!"

"Is his name Bob?" asked Derrick, who had strolled in.

"Well, yes," said Lynda, looking perplexed.

"Is he from B.C.?" he asked.

"Yeah." She suddenly clued in. "Derrick, FUCK OFF!"

With that, she stormed back to her console. Although Ali repeatedly tried to fool her with a fake Iranian accent after that ("Ali, I know that's you." Click.), Lynda never fell for that gag again.

The crew Lynda ended up booking was all freelancers that

Electric Images had used on other shows. They were all young, in their 20s or early 30s, and most of them had grown up listening to the *Sunday Night Sex Show* on the radio.

Sana was asked to get together with Sue before the first episode and go over make-up and clothing. She remembers their first contact: "I had heard her on the radio, coming back from the cottage or whatever, but when I heard her voice on my answering machine, I thought 'Oh my God!' It's such a distinctive voice. It was exciting."

When they met, her impression was that Sue would be easy to get along with. "She was easy to please," Sana confesses. And she was, until the notorious "Hair Incident."

For several episodes, Sana undertook the laborious task of straightening Sue's curls. This involved a curling iron and a considerable amount of time. Sue ended up with a classic, coifed look that, frankly, made her look quite glamorous. But, not knowing Sue's long history of hair tribulations, Sana's efforts were the equivalent of poking a pit bull until it woke up. Then, one Sunday, the jaws snapped.

"I pulled out the curling iron," says Sana, "and Sue looked at me and said, 'You're not doing it. You're just not going to do it to me.' I said, 'Julie's going to be really upset.' And she said, 'Well, I guess we're going to Julie then.' Julie *was* really upset, but Sue wouldn't back down. I've never seen her put her foot down as strongly about anything else," she pauses. "Except maybe circumcision."

Episode One of the *Sunday Night Sex Show* aired on WTN at 10:30 Eastern time on February 4, 1996. As with any new show, the Control Room was thick with tension. Since the show had started an hour earlier on radio, Lynda already had calls lined up for the television broadcast. Julie, who had never produced a live program in her life, was nearly catatonic with fear.

"I was petrified, absolutely petrified. I can remember, I didn't know what I was doing then. I was just kind of sitting there. The first call went to air and it was all sort of working."

The way the phone system was set up, Julie had to push the button that actually sent the call to air. She and Lynda quickly discovered that if the button was held down, rather than pushed, it dumped all 10 calls on hold. I vaguely remember some panicked hollering about this from the back of the Control Room. ("Shit! We've lost all our calls! Get Sue to do a letter!")

Just before the program started, Chris entered the studio to do a last minute check of Sue's IFB. He remembers that she was so scared, she was shaking.

"I couldn't believe that, after all those years of doing the cable show, she was so nervous about it," he says. "Because this was a national show, it was a huge step for her. I remember taking her hand and saying, 'Relax. It's just TV,' and her hand was freezing."

Aside from fear, Sue had her own technical challenges. She is generally befuddled by any technology more complex than a Singer sewing machine. On the first show, she didn't quite understand the segue between the radio portion and the television portion. In her confusion, she read the television introduction, which explained what the new program was all about and her background, while the opening animation was

running. So, by the time the viewer saw her, she was just getting to, "Okay, let's take another call." Of course, viewers were
left scratching their heads. "Another call? But haven't you just
started?" As Sue is quick to point out, it wasn't the last time
she left viewers baffled.

There was also the problem of the cock-ring.

In the pre-production meeting, Julie and I had gone
through the props that Sue wanted to have on the set for reference: a diaphragm, a condom, some lubricant, her jointed
dollies for showing sexual positions, a wood dildo, and so on.

"What's this?" Julie held up a small rubber ring, about two
inches wide. It looked more suitable for canning preserves.

"It's a cock-ring," explained Sue. "If a male is having trouble maintaining an erection, you stretch this over the base of
the penis and it holds the blood in."

"Sue, you can't say 'cock-ring' on air," Julie stated firmly.

Sue protested, "Julie, there's no other name for it. That's
what it's called."

"Can't you say 'penis-ring' instead?"

Sue considered a moment. "Yeah, okay, I'll say 'penis-ring'
if it comes up."

A week later, on the second episode, it did. A caller had a
question about keeping his erection. Sure enough, Sue
retrieved it from her props, held it up in front of her, and pro-
claimed, "Here's what you need. A cock-ring!"

Julie howled "No!" from the back of the Control Room as
Sue blithely explained to the caller how to stretch the cock-
ring around a penis, pull it down to the base, and not leave it
on too long. She probably said the forbidden word half a
dozen times.

"I don't think I slept at all that night," chuckles Julie. "I thought for sure the CRTC was going to take us off the air the very next day. Nobody else was doing anything this 'out there' on Canadian television at the time. So, I got to work the next day, and there were no phone calls waiting for me. I waited. Still no calls. And, I thought, 'Oh, okay . . . cock-ring it is!'"

During the first episode, Susan Millican was having her own nightmare. She had taken a huge gamble by committing to such an explicit program, and had flown to Toronto to attend its launch. However, when she reached the studio, the doors were locked and there was no intercom to the Control Room. She went into a bar next door and asked the bartender to switch the giant TV screen to WTN so she could catch the premiere. With all the guys in the bar watching, Susan repeatedly used her cell phone, trying to contact Julie. The guys, of course, assumed that she had an urgent sexual problem that could only be addressed by Sue. Finally, she was rescued. I remember her coming into the Control Room about halfway through the show, looking no less nervous than the rest of us.

Susan undoubtedly relaxed the next day when she saw the ratings — the very first episode had drawn 100,000 viewers. For the next six seasons, the *Sunday Night Sex Show* remained WTN's highest-rated Canadian production, averaging between 200,000 and 300,000 viewers every week.

With the first 13 episodes a ratings success, the show was picked up for a second season of 26 shows. Although Sue was, and is, the main attraction, Julie's contribution was no less crucial. Chris Priess observes: "Right from the start I could see how much the show meant to Julie. She took a controversial local show and made it into an acceptable national show by guiding Sue along." Shanda Deziel adds, "It was just as much Julie. She made Sue TV-friendly."

In the middle of the second season, we moved to a new facility, Electric Entertainment on Jarvis Street, in the heart of downtown.

This proved to be a more appropriate location for a show about sex, since we were suddenly surrounded by hookers and pimps. The tiny, poorly-lit parking lot behind the building was frequently littered with used condoms. The recessed doorway at the side, which we used as an entrance, stank of piss. At first, the newly renovated interior was pristine, but that deteriorated during the two-and-a-half years we were at the facility. One winter, a family of pigeons took up residence in the studio's exhaust fan. Luckily, they sleep at night — during the taping of another daytime show, one flew over the set and shit on a host.

Getting in and out of the parking lot through the narrow laneway beside Electric Entertainment was particularly difficult in the winter, especially for Sue, who is not always the best with spatial perception. Shanda hitched a harrowing ride on several occasions: "I was scared to get in the car with Sue because I think she hit something in that driveway every time. One time I was there, she hit the wall with her passenger's side rearview mirror, and broke it right off. I was sitting right there, thinking, 'Oh my God, she's going to ram into this wall!'" She did.

One other notable incident occurred at Electric Entertainment. In this case, what happened remains a mystery.

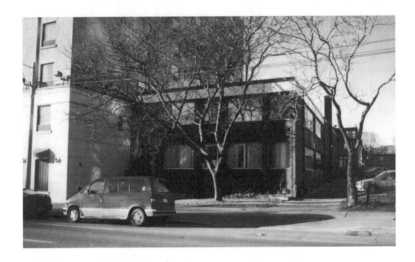

Electric Entertainment Studio

We were set up to do an episode. The feed to Winnipeg had been checked 30 minutes before air-time. Ten minutes before the broadcast, the connection vanished. The technical producer and engineer scrambled madly, searching for the problem. They checked with Bell to make sure the output was being fed to Winnipeg. It was. We warned Master Control to stand by with a repeat show. At one minute to air, which is my cut-off time for a live broadcast, we instructed them to run the repeat. We carried on in the Control Room and studio as if we were doing a live show, and simply taped it for future airing. Viewers watching the repeat program continued to call in as if it were live, and we didn't tell Sue we weren't — there was no point throwing her off. Halfway through the production, the problem was discovered — someone had purposely severed the feed-line in the rear of the building. No other lines were cut. The phones and power were left intact. Whoever chopped the feed knew exactly what he or she was doing, and would have required a heavy duty bolt-cutter to do it. Many people object to the program on moral grounds and this may have been the motivation; but, to this day, we have never uncovered the truth. We suspect Dr. Ruth.

♀♂

The relocation to SkyDome was a welcome change, beer barrels notwithstanding. As with the previous move, Julie refused to go without the crew.

"It was part of the deal that we could bring whoever we wanted with us, our key people, to that new studio" says Julie. "We were insistent, as a family, that we would not even consider moving to another facility without being able to bring our family with us."

Dome Productions was reluctant at first, since they had their own roster of freelancers. Ultimately, they relented. Now they book members of our crew for their own productions.

Ivan Kosir joined the crew as our videotape operator when we moved to SkyDome. It didn't take him long to suffer "The Curse" of the *Sunday Night Sex Show*.

During our first season, the show aired a half-hour earlier than it does currently, and we were more inclined to go out for a beer together after the broadcast. Near the end of that season, we were at the local pub and someone pointed out that, since they'd been working on the show, they hadn't gotten laid once. Comparing notes, we discovered that, to our dismay,

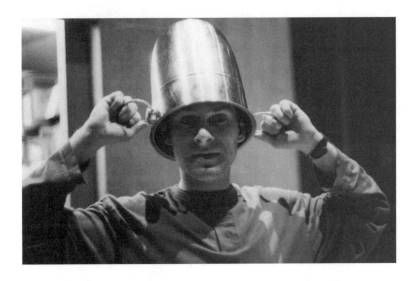

Ivan demonstrates the requisite equipment for working in the television industry. (Photo courtesy Ali Miraliakbari)

none of us had had any sex since the show started. This was dubbed "The Curse."

Ivan admits, "Julie warned me about 'The Curse.' I think people on the show just know too much about sex. It scares girls off. They find it intimidating."

"It's so true!" says Shanda. "Those first two years, I didn't see anybody. My Dad would say, 'Well, no man is going to sleep with you now. They'll be all worried about what you know and what you're judging. It's threatening that you work on a sex show.' Thank you, Dad!"

"The Curse" affected Lynda and Julie in an altogether different way. While Sue was answering questions about genital warts, herpes, chlamydia, yeast infections, HIV, gonorrhoea, and all manner of sexual distress, they were getting more and more grossed out by the idea of ever having sex again. "I remember asking Sue if a guy could wear six condoms at once!" laughs Julie. "It took the first season to get over that."

♀♂

To the uninitiated, the term "control room" seems like a misnomer. The "out-of-control room" would be a more suitable appellation for the pandemonium that appears to reign there during a live broadcast. The constant drone of on-air chatter, the raised voices demanding immediate action, the perpetual countdown, the jibes, the hoots, the hollers, the threats, all tinged with a patina of edgy panic — it's a tidal wave of chaos to the outsider. Yet, shows get on the air and workers go home with a sliver of sanity intact, so the system somehow works.

Most people are on headsets and the secret is to sort out what you need to hear and what you don't need to hear. Just be thankful none of us are driving while we're doing this.

The phone calls generally last three minutes, depending on the complexity of the problem and Sue's answer. Regardless, the production assistant counts three minutes for each call and I extend the time if it's required. Except for the last segment, if a call runs long — and they frequently do — we can recover the time by dropping a call later in the show.

Trying to understand what goes on in the Control Room could be a three-year course at Centennial College. The next few pages offer a much shorter road to wisdom with my "Simultaneity Sampler." These are fictional calls and times, but they'll give you some idea of how the pieces of the puzzle fit together.

TIME	ON AIR
11:17:00	SUE: [turning to Camera 1] We've got Sarah on the line. Hello Sarah?
	SARAH: Hi Sue. How are you?
	SUE: I'm just fine. You got a question?
	SARAH: I've just started dating a new boyfriend and the other night we had sexual relations for the first time.
	SUE: Okay.
	SARAH: Well, the problem is that his penis has a huge bend in it. I've never seen one like that before.
	SUE: And did you have sexual intercourse?
	SARAH: Yes.
11:17:30	SUE: And did the bend in his penis make intercourse painful or uncomfortable for you?
	SARAH: Well, a little bit. Is there anything he can do about it, like straighten it?
	SUE: He has something called Peyronie's disease. A lot of males have a curved penis and it's caused by an injury that happened when they were just little boys. They could have been hit in the groin with a hockey stick, or a puck, or a baseball, and what actually happens is that their penis gets injured. [Sue reaches for her wooden penis] Tissue gets damaged on one side of the penis and scar tissue forms. [She demonstrates on
11:18:00	model] Since scar tissue doesn't expand like the regular

CONTROL ROOM	CALL SCREENING
R.J.: [To Sue's IFB] Take Camera 1	MONA: *Sunday Night Sex Show.* Can I have your name please? CALLER: Michelle.
R.J.: [to Liisa and Liz] Stand by name super. LIISA: Standing by. R.J.: [to Liz] Super in. [Liz adds super — "Sarah/Chilliwack"]	MONA: Michelle, where are you calling from? CALLER: Windsor. MONA: And what's your question for Sue? CALLER: One of my nipples is bleeding.
R.J.: Super out. [Liz pulls it out]	MONA: Have you seen your doctor about this? CALLER: No, not yet.
WHOLE CONTROL ROOM: Peyronie's!	MONA: And how long has it been bleeding? [She looks at Julie, who cringes] CALLER: Since Friday. MONA: Michelle, this sounds like a medical problem and Sue is not a doctor. I'm not going to put you on air, but would you make an appointment to see your family doctor tomorrow? CALLER: Okay. MONA: Good. Thanks for calling the *Sunday Night Sex Show.* [Takes next call] *Sunday Night Sex Show.* Can I have your name please?
R.J.: Germain, loosen up a bit. [Germain zooms back to show Sue and penis] LIISA: [To all] Two minutes left in call.	CALLER: Wilma. MONA: Wilma, where are you calling from?

TIME	ON AIR
	spongy tissue in a penis, it causes it to pull to one side. That's what makes it curve.
	SARAH: I see.
	SUE: Trying to straighten it out is a whole other story. You can't really put some heavy cookbooks, or encyclopedias, or *anything* on it and leave it overnight. Won't work. Often in younger guys, the problem resolves itself and the scar tissue dissolves on its own. I know they've done some tests with Vitamin E and with collagen injections, but so far there's nothing conclusive about using those as a
11:18:30	treatment. In drastic cases, a doctor can perform a surgery and remove the scar tissue, which will straighten the penis out, or make it somewhat straighter. The problem with that is that any surgery on the penis can cause nerve damage that may be permanent. How bent is it?
	SARAH: I'd say almost a 90-degree bend.
	SUE: Woah! That's pretty extreme. Maybe you could suggest to him that he talk to his family doctor about it. Did you tell him it was uncomfortable?
11:19:00	SARAH: No. I didn't want to hurt his feelings.
	SUE: Sarah, honey, look — you may not want to hurt his feelings, but the alternative is him physically hurting you. That's not a very good trade-off, is it?

CONTROL ROOM	CALL SCREENING
R.J.: [To Julie] Julie, how are the calls? [To Liisa] Pull up the graphic of the erect penis in case Sue wants to use it. LIISA: [Finds graphic] Got it. R.J.: [To Julie] We'll put up the phone number. [To Liisa and Liz] Standby phone super. LIISA: Standing by. R.J.: Super in. [Liz dissolves phone number super in] R.J.: [To Sue's IFB] Got a graphic if you want it. [Sue shakes her head 'No' while talking on air.]	JULIE: [To R.J.] A bit slow at the moment. CALLER: Bedrock. MONA: And what's your question for Sue? JULIE: [To R.J.] Good idea. CALLER: How can I tell if my husband is having an affair? MONA: Are you concerned that he is? CALLER: Yes. MONA: What makes you think so? CALLER: He seems to spend a lot of time away from home with our next door neighbour, Barney. They say they're going bowling. MONA: And do you suspect that they are having a relationship?
R.J.: Super out. [Liz pulls it] LIISA: [To all] One minute. R.J.: [To Sue's IFB] One minute.	CALLER: I'm starting to wonder. MONA: So, Wilma, your concern is that your husband is having a same-sex affair, is that right? [She nudges Julie] CALLER: Yes. MONA: Wilma, I'm just going to put you on hold a moment. [Puts caller on hold and turns to Julie] I've got a woman here who thinks her husband is having an affair with his best friend, a guy.

TIME	ON AIR
	SARAH: No.
	SUE: Are you hoping this is going to turn into a long-term relationship?
	SARAH: Yes, I hope so, but this sort of puts me off.
	SUE: I can see how it would if intercourse is going to be painful every time you have sex. How would you
11:19:30	feel about approaching him about it? You know, do it gently and do it while you're washing dishes, or driving, or doing something other than lying in bed together. How would you feel about that?
	SARAH: I guess I could do that.
	SUE: I think if he wants to get serious about the relationship, then he'll listen to you and maybe take some action. Otherwise, he's going to spend a whole lotta time playing with himself. Okay, Sarah?
	SARAH: Okay. Thanks Sue.
11:20:00	SUE: Thank you and good luck. Bye bye. Now it's on to Wilma in Bedrock.

CONTROL ROOM	CALL SCREENING
	JULIE: Can she talk?
	MONA: Yeah, she's well-spoken.
	JULIE: That's probably a more common prob-
	lem than people think. Let's put her on next.
LIISA: [To all] 30 seconds.	MONA: [To caller] Hi Wilma. The producer
R.J.: [To Sue's IFB] Wrap it up.	feels that this would be a good call for Sue to
	answer. Can you hold on a few minutes?
	JULIE: [To all] Our next caller is Wilma from
	Bedrock. That's Wilma from Bedrock. Got
LIISA: [To Julie] Got it. [She starts typ-	that?
ing name into character generator]	CALLER: Yes.
ALI: [From studio] Got it. [He starts	MONA: When you tell Sue your story, do
typing name into prompter]	not mention any names. Okay?
R.J.: [To all] She's wrapping up. Standby	CALLER: Okay, I won't.
Camera 1.	MONA: Okay, I'm putting you on hold. You will
R.J.: [To all] Standby Camera 1.	hear Sue next. [Puts caller on hold] *Sunday*
R.J.: [To Sue's IFB] Take 1.	*Night Sex Show.* Can I have your name please?
	CALLER: Betty.
	MONA: And where are you calling from,
	Betty?

The *Sunday Night Sex Show* has the simplest format imaginable. It's essentially a radio show with pictures. Think about what a sampler would look like for three minutes of a hockey game — with dozens of camera cuts, taped replays, and multiple supers. Suddenly, those instructions for putting the gas barbecue together seem downright elementary.

The toughest part of the program is the last segment. Before the show, Sue rehearses her book review and closing while Liisa times it. So, going into the last segment, we know how much time that will take, plus we know the length of the closing credits. Liisa subtracts that amount from the out-time of the show, and, during the last commercial break, we tell Sue

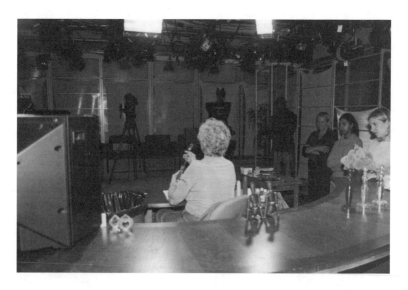

A shot from behind the set. Sue rehearses with a toy while Liisa, Priya, and Julie consider the possibilities.

how much time she has left for calls. When we hit the book review, I'm usually whispering sweet nothings in her ear ("Stretch," "Speed it up") and she follows my instructions accordingly. Of course, this results in a peripatetic speech pattern that must leave viewers wondering whether or not Sue is having a seizure.

Miraculously, it all works and comes out on time. Dwayne rolls the closing theme, which Sue can hear, and that's her cue to wrap it up, and fast. She always ends with a signature "condom closer," a humorous line she's come up with that reinforces the practice of safer sex. Liisa rolls the credits. I watch the off-air monitor until I see the final credit roll by, and the next show start on WTN.

The studio guys strike the set, the dildos get put away, the last of the sourdough biscuits gets eaten, and we're off into the night, way too tired to have any sex ourselves.

Sue's Opening Remarks

Viewers may have missed Sue's opening remarks on the first episode of the *Sunday Night Sex Show* because of Sue's gaffe — but here they are, from the original script:

"Welcome to the *Sunday Night Sex Show*. If you have a question, a concern, problems in your relationship, difficulties communicating or establishing intimacy, let's talk. Call me, toll free, 1-800-881-5514.

Some of you may not know me. Since 1984, I have been the host of the *Sunday Night Sex Show* on RADIO AM 640 which is heard in many cities right across Canada. I have also written three books: *Talk Sex, Sex Is Perfectly Natural, But Not Naturally Perfect.* Last spring, *Sex, Sex and More Sex* was published. I also write a weekly column for the Edmonton *Sun*.

In addition, I do presentations at universities, community colleges, and senior high schools right across Canada.

As host of *Talking Sex* on Rogers Cable TV in Southern Ontario for 11 years, I had the dream of doing a national TV show for all Canadians. This is it. So give us a call."

Dink Don't Work

Seemingly, many Canadians who own telephones also have sexual problems.

The average episode of the *Sunday Night Sex Show* receives 65,000 attempted calls. Of those, 50 to 100 get through to the call screener, and only 12 to 16 make it to air. If Sue talked with every single caller for an average of three minutes each, it would take her 135 days to respond to all the calls generated by one episode.

Based on the number of calls, Edmonton led the way as "Sexual Dysfunction Capital of Canada" for the first three seasons, but that flaccid honour has since passed to St. John's, Newfoundland.

The most frequently asked question is (drum roll) "Where's my G-spot?" Mona receives several of these each night, but we only air one every few weeks to avoid being repetitive. Instead, callers are urged to write in and receive Sue's print-out on locating the almighty G-spot, which is apparently better hidden than King Solomon's mines.

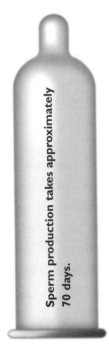

Sperm production takes approximately 70 days.

Right from the start, Sue told Julie that there were three topics she wouldn't deal with: bestiality, paedophilia, and necrophilia. In the first season, Julie played it safe by sticking with the most basic questions, such as erectile dysfunction, pregnancy, and yeast infections. However, Sue's responses to yeast-infection calls ("What colour is the discharge? Is it clear and oozy, or green and slimy like snot? Is it odourless or does it smell like a wharf in Dartmouth?") soon put "pus" on the VERBOTEN list.

Julie says, "Pus became my pet peeve because of how explicit Sue would get. It would turn my stomach, so I figured viewers were having the same reaction."

Pus is not the topic that viewers complain about the most, however. The subject that consistently gets the biggest negative reaction is whenever Sue suggests to a lesbian caller who wants to become pregnant that she simply use a turkey-baster for impregnation. The mere mention of this method — a tried and true squirt, by the way — drives viewers absolutely wacky. Men are offended at the suggestion that they can be replaced by a kitchen utensil, and women are offended thinking about next Thanksgiving.

As the population is ageing, we get more and more calls about erectile dysfunction, sometimes from a man, but more often from his concerned partner. This problem can have a number of different causes, so it frequently makes it to air. In fact, we've developed a Control Room acronym to indicate when that type of call is coming up: D.D.W., or "Dink Don't Work." It lets us know which graphics may be required. ("Got a D.D.W. call next. Have the 'penis without erection' graphic standing by.")

Julie and Mona ride herd on the line-up of calls, and I

occasionally throw in my two cents' worth. After many years of doing this, I know how long it will take Sue to answer a particular question (painful urination: four minutes; dink too small: two minutes) and, being in the front line, I know how much time we have to fill.

The phones start ringing about half an hour before the show begins. As Mona weeds out the keepers, she enters the pertinent information into a computer stationed at her post. It displays the caller's name, location, and a brief description of the question. That display appears in front of Liisa, Dwayne, Ali, and me. It shows all 10 calls on hold, but not their order of appearance, which is why Julie conveys that information by headset. Sometimes people will be on hold for an hour, and then have their call dumped when a previous caller asks their same question spontaneously. Mona apologizes profusely, but she's been sworn at by callers many, many times. None of us enjoy pissing off viewers, but the show has to be entertaining as well as educational, and, in the immortal words of Celine Dion, "dat's da way it is." They can always write to Sue.

Julie and Mona have a specific set of criteria that they're looking for in phone calls: "We're looking for things that we haven't covered recently," Julie says. "We want diversity in the questions, and if we dealt with a subject that was odd the week before, we don't want that same subject two weeks in a row. We try to get a mix of male and female calls, and calls from different areas of the country." They also look for people who are well-spoken, although, when Lynda was doing the call-screening, she would fight for a weak talker if she felt the question was compelling. She says, "Julie usually had enough confidence in my judgement to use the call. If I screwed up, though, and the call sucked, it would take a few weeks before she'd trust me again."

Of course, this begs the obvious question: What kind of person would phone into a television show with a personal problem?

"There are two types," says Sue, "the ones who just want to hear themselves on air, and the ones who are desperate. They really feel they have nowhere else to turn. Often they just want reassurance that they're 'normal' or that their feelings are valid. I tell them to listen to their gut. It already has the answer."

After the caller gets on air, I take over and determine the length of the call. Liisa counts the standard three minutes, but I don't relay that to Sue. I just listen and go by my gut. If it's interesting, I let it go, sometimes up to five minutes. If it's not holding my attention, I give Sue a 30-second cue in her IFB, and she wraps it up. Dwayne and I are both very attuned to callers, and have a natural "sixth sense" about potential trouble. If we feel a caller is about to go off the rails, either by swearing or asking another question, we pull him or her down. The caller can still hear Sue, but she can't hear them. I tell Sue "Caller pulled" in her IFB, and she understands why they're not responding to her.

We use the IFB judiciously. It's quite confusing to have another voice talking in your ear while *you're* talking, so I try to use it as little as possible. If Sue misunderstands a call, I'll simply say, "Ask again." That lets her know that she's on the wrong track. Some callers, which we refer to as "yeah, but" callers, have no solution to their problem because, every time Sue proposes one, they say, "Yeah, but . . ." and come up with another excuse. These calls can turn into an endless spiral with

Sue making one suggestion after another. Finally, I say "No answer" in her earpiece, and we drop the call.

Although Sue appears to be totally focused on each caller and unconcerned about the rest of the audience, she is always conscious of not offending people, including the religious right.

"I'm very, very non-judgmental, and many of them are very critical. I'm conscious of the religious right because I don't want to offend them. I'm not placating them, but I'm concerned about offending them. I don't want to alienate them because, usually, their attitudes stem from lack of information, a lack of knowledge. If we can get that knowledge through, you know. . . . More is accomplished by sugar than by vinegar."

♀♂

Although Sue Johanson is the star of the show, the callers are the co-stars. Some calls have made us laugh and some calls have been deeply upsetting. Rarely is a person's problem unique and, for the one person who phones in, dozens of others may be helped by hearing Sue's answer.

I asked the gang to recall some of their favourite phone calls from the past six seasons, questions that were unusual or funny or that touched them somehow. I've changed the name and location of callers to protect their privacy and compressed some dialogue, but the gist of the query is still intact.

My favourite phone call didn't even get on air. It didn't get past Mona, but I thought it was especially cute:

MONA: *Sunday Night Sex Show.* Where are you calling from?

CALLER: (young boy whispers) My bedroom.

MONA: (more determined) And where's that?

CALLER: (whispers) The second floor.

At which point, Mona hit the "Hold" button and dissolved into laughter. This young kid was obviously watching the show in his bedroom and didn't want his parents to know. I don't remember what his question was, but this sweet incident is symbolic of the breadth of the show's appeal and the trust that viewers of all ages have in Sue.

So, welcome to the *Sunday Night Sex Show!*

> One female in 1000 is born
> without a uterus.

Smooth or Crunchy?

SUE: Carl is calling from Halifax. Hi Carl. Got a question?

CARL: Hi Sue. My question is — I like to have sex with different objects, like a peanut butter jar for instance.

SUE: A peanut butter what?

CARL: A jar of peanut butter.

SUE: Right.

CARL: Because I don't get a lot of sex. The girls in my grade don't want to have sex with me, so I try to do it with different things.

SUE: So you're sticking your penis into a jar of peanut butter?

CARL: Yes, I stick my penis in.

SUE: Okay (starts to giggle).

CARL: I just want to know if that's dangerous or not.

SUE: No. You know what? Cleaning up would be such a sticky mess that I would be inclined to wear a condom.

CARL: Oh! That's a good idea.

SUE: You would be protecting yourself, and, I was going to say, protecting the peanut butter, but that doesn't make any sense. Peanut butter is fine, no problem.

CARL: What about other things, like vegetables?

SUE: What? You're going to stick your penis into what? Squash?

CARL: You know, you cut them open to make them look like a vagina.

SUE: (pauses) That takes a real leap of faith to imagine that a turnip looks like a vagina. It *has* been a long time since you've had sex.

CARL: Yeah, I've only had sex a couple of times.

SUE: What about ordinary masturbation?

CARL: (exasperated) It just doesn't cut it anymore. I masturbate a lot, like three or four times a day.

SUE: I can see how that would get boring, but what you do is develop different fantasies so you're not just flipping into the same one over and over.

CARL: Oh, okay.

SUE: But the peanut butter is fine. Just don't put it back in the cupboard when you're done.

Food may be the way to a man's heart, but it also appears to be a popular sexual object. Barely a show goes by without someone asking a question about inserting something edible into their orifices. I swear, we get more food questions than a cooking show. Maybe we should just book Bonnie Stern on, and be done with it.

Oh, Henry!

SUE: We've got Joyce from Antigonish on the line. Hi Joyce. Got a question?

JOYCE: Hi Sue. My husband and I want to experiment.

SUE: Uh, huh.

JOYCE: We want to try inserting a chocolate bar into my vagina.

SUE: (grimaces) Not a great idea. Chocolate is very, very sweet and the sugar will change the acid/alkaline balance of your vagina, which can contribute to a nasty yeast infection.

JOYCE: Oh, I'm glad I didn't do it.

SUE: No, chocolate is not a great idea. Marshmallows, not a great idea. A popsicle, not a great idea. If you want to try a small zucchini or a carrot that's washed, you can do that. But nothing that's really, really sweet.

JOYCE: I tried a cucumber once but forgot to wash it.

SUE: Did you get a yeast infection?

JOYCE: No.

SUE: Well, you're probably not going to get yeast from a cucumber. It's just the idea of putting mud in your vagina that leaves something to be desired. Wash it first.

I Can't Hear You . . . Part One

SUE: And we've got Marie from Calgary on the line. Hi Marie, how are you?

MARIE: I'm not doing so great.

SUE: Why, what's the matter?

MARIE: Well, I'm a regular viewer and my boyfriend and I like to watch your show. We were watching your show before, when you said you could use fruit or stuff like that. So, we were using a banana and part of the banana broke off and now it's lodged in there and we can't seem to get it out.

SUE: (chuckles) Okay, so it's up in your vagina?

MARIE: Yes, it's stuck there.

SUE: What you may have to do is actually wash it out. The easiest way to do that would be with a douche. Have you got a douche nozzle?

MARIE: No, but we could go and buy one tomorrow. Can we wait that long?

SUE: Hey, Marie, why don't you go and have a long bath, not a bubble bath, just an ordinary bath, okay? Now you're in the water, you're submerged in the water, you take one or two fingers, put it in your vagina — this is okay, nothing bad is going to happen — just reach in your vagina and pull out the pieces of banana.

MARIE: You think the bath will relax me enough for the banana to come out?

SUE: Oh sure, the water will swish in and wash out the vagina and you'll probably be fine. I wouldn't worry about it too much.

MARIE: Great. Thanks Sue. We'll try that right now (she hangs up).

SUE: I think the advice was to leave the skin on the banana but, hey, who am I to say?

♀♂

One call that made us howl concerned anal intercourse, but we were laughing at Sue's faux pas, not at the caller. The woman had asked what type of vibrator would be safe for anal penetration. Sue was suggesting a slender, flexible device called "The Wild Thing." She innocently demonstrated its width by holding up her middle finger in a classic "third finger salute." I had been looking down at the line-up and when I looked up, there she was, giving 300,000 viewers the finger. And it wasn't a brief gesture — she sat there for at least 10 seconds making her point. When we went to break, we told her what she had done, and she roared with laughter. After the break, she apologized to viewers, commenting that if it was good enough for Pierre Elliott Trudeau, it was good enough for her.

> During sexual intercourse, the average male thrusts from 60 to 120 times before ejaculation.

Anatomy 101

SUE: We've got Roger on the phone from Winnipeg. Hi Roger. Got a question?

ROGER: I was wondering if my partner could become pregnant from oral sex.

SUE: No.

ROGER: So, no, it's not possible.

SUE: So what you're saying is that your partner performs oral sex on you?

ROGER: Yes, and she's worried that she could become pregnant if I ejaculate down her throat.

SUE: The digestive system and the reproductive system are two entirely separate systems. If she eats a peanut butter and jam sandwich, does it end up in her vagina?

ROGER: No.

SUE: So no, there's no way.

Shanda Deziel says, "One of the things I admire about Sue is that she treats each question as if she's never heard it before, even if she's answered it a million times."

"Every question is valid," says Sue, "and that's the whole point of the show. I never think someone is stupid for asking a question, but sometimes I am bewildered, more than anything, that they don't have that knowledge already. The calls I have the most trouble with are where someone is having an affair with somebody else who's married. Not from a moral standpoint, not that at all. Women will have an affair with a married man in the hopes that he will marry them, and I heard statistics that less than 10 percent ever marry. They're just deluding themselves. Also I'm concerned that the partner who is having the affair can bring home diseases and put his marriage partner at risk. Sometimes, I can get judgemental and even get downright angry."

Not a Nice Lady

SUE: Up next, we've got Michelle. Hi Michelle.

MICHELLE: Hi Sue. I've got a problem. During foreplay, my boyfriend has this really bad habit of biting me during oral sex. I would like to talk to him about it but I don't want to hurt his feelings and it's going too far.

SUE: (mouth open in shock) He does *what* to you?

MICHELLE: He bites me.

SUE: Oh . . . ouch! You just want to get out of that situation. It hurts! Because when you're turned on, your genitals are super sensitive.

MICHELLE: I'm not exactly sure of how to get him to stop.

SUE: Gee whiz, I have to say, I'm not a nice lady. He'd be getting a smart whack on the side of the head . . . (makes slapping motion). That's not nice, I shouldn't have said it. But it would certainly get his attention, wouldn't it?

MICHELLE: Yeah, I guess so, but I don't want to hurt his feelings.

SUE: Wait a minute!! Why are we worried about his feelings when he is hurting you? Hello??

MICHELLE: Right.

SUE: Why are we pussyfooting around, and scared of hurting his feelings when he is physically abusing you? Hurt his feelings — trample on them! I told you I wasn't a nice lady. What if you bit him?

MICHELLE: (laughs) Maybe I should.

SUE: Well, that's one thing I wouldn't do, and there's not much I wouldn't do, but I wouldn't do that because he might like it and then we're in deep doo-doo. So I would give him an ultimatum — you do that again, buster, and we're finished. Don't do that again, it hurts. Read my lips. Forget his feelings on this one. If he wants to chew on something, get him a Milk-Bone.

Return for Deposit

SUE: And now we've got Claire from Montreal. Hello Claire. What's your question?

CLAIRE: My boyfriend likes to have sex with me with objects, odd ones, like beer bottles and bike locks and stuff like that. Is that okay?

SUE: (appalled) I would say not! Certain things are okay, but not glass. Why do we want to have beer bottles?

CLAIRE: It's anything, like bike locks, beer bottles, and candles, stuff like that.

SUE: And you don't like this?

CLAIRE: No, I don't.

SUE: You need to tell him.

CLAIRE: Well, I tried, but it's one of those things where he's really keen on it and I really don't know what to say.

SUE: (peeved) Well, that's unfortunate that he's really *keen* on it because you're not. It's turning you right off. The minute he looks at a beer bottle you're going to say to him, "Don't even think about it."

CLAIRE: Yeah, when we do go to parties I'm really uncomfortable.

SUE: Tell him your vagina is not designed for beer bottles or candles and, "It's not what I want. If that's what *you* want, then I'm sorry, we are not going to be able to make this relationship work." Claire, this is a form of abuse that he's forcing on you with intimidation. It's *your* body and it's time you take charge.

During arousal, the testicles increase approximately 50 percent from their unstimulated size.

The Incredible Shrinking Woman

SUE: We've got Dawn on the line from Sudbury. Hi Dawn — got a question?

DAWN: My boyfriend's in the Navy and he goes out for a few months at a time. Every time he comes out, he says I should be smaller when he gets back. He has no reason to think that I cheat on him or anything.

SUE: Does he think that you shrink?

DAWN: Yeah, like I told him I don't think that's possible.

SUE: Ask him if he shrinks. This is anatomically impossible. This guy doesn't know from nothing. Don't you let him upset you. There is no way — the vagina does not shrink or atrophy or shrivel up until you are about 90 years of age.

DAWN: He says that I should be tighter, like if I'm not having sex or anything.

SUE: Does he think that if you don't drive the car there'll be more gas in the tank next time?

DAWN: Probably.

SUE: What he says you should be is not the way you are, and you tell him that if he wants you tighter, it ain't going to work and he gotta go and find somebody else. Okay, Dawn?

DAWN: Thanks Sue.

One thing we've discovered is that Canadians are generous with advice. If someone calls with a problem that's out of the ordinary, another person will inevitably call the next week with the same problem and a solution. We love when this happens because it truly makes the program what it should be, a forum about sexuality and relationships for everyone.

What's Taking You So Long in There? Part One

SUE: And now we've got Jan from Windsor on the line. Hi Jan.

JAN: Hi Sue. My husband has a strange problem.

SUE: Okay.

JAN: When he's in the bathroom and he strains for a bowel movement, he ejaculates.

SUE: (looks puzzled)

JAN: He asked his doctor and his doctor said it's very normal. It happens about once a month. Should he be concerned?

SUE: (scratching her head) Jan, I have never heard this in my life. You're going to have to let me ask my resident experts and get back to you on next week's show.

JAN: Okay.

SUE: Relax. Nothing bad is going to happen. He's not going to explode or anything like that.

[One Week Later . . .]

SUE: We've got Ken from Saskatoon next. Hi Ken.

KEN: Hi Sue. I want to respond to that girl's call from last week about her husband who ejaculates when he goes for a bowel movement.

SUE: Yes!

KEN: Something like that has been happening to me since I was around 15. It's not like a full ejaculation.

SUE: Oh.

KEN: There's just a small amount of ejaculate.

SUE: Is it like lubrication, you know, the clear liquid, or is it white and thick?

KEN: Occasionally, it is just lubrication, but usually, it's the actual ejaculate — milky white.

SUE: (shakes her head) Well, I'm wondering if faeces coming down your bowel stimulates the prostate gland.

KEN: Well, it could have something to do with the amount of muscle flexing you do in that area as well, when you're really straining.

SUE: Alright, I couldn't find anything out about this, but I'm going to have to go back to the drawing board again.

[Another Week Later . . .]

SUE: I got my call-backs from my doctors, and they said it's not unusual for a male, sitting on the john, there's vasoconstriction around the tush and that blood collects in the genitals, and it's not unusual for him to have an erection. He may even lubricate. It would be the thick, clear mucous secretion. But, for him to ejaculate, it would be quite unusual. So, if it's happening for him, there's no problem at all and he should enjoy having a bowel movement. Hey, at least the toilet paper is handy!

What's Taking You So Long in There? Part Two

SUE: And now we've got Frank on the phone from Moose Jaw. Hi Frank.

FRANK: Could you tell me, sometimes when I'm urinating, at the end when I'm trying to eliminate the last drop, I'll actually have ejaculate come out.

SUE: Are you sure it's ejaculate?

FRANK: Yes.

SUE: What makes you sure?

FRANK: Just the consistency, the difference in the sensation as it travels . . .

SUE: So you're standing up to urinate. I've had the question before from males sitting down and ejaculating when they're having a bowel movement, but I've never had the question from somebody standing up urinating and ejaculating that way. I want to be sure it's ejaculate, because if it's thick and kind of a white colour, I worry about a sexually transmitted disease. Is that possible?

FRANK: Not to my knowledge.

SUE: There's no burning sensation?

FRANK: No.

SUE: So when you're urinating it doesn't feel like somebody stuck a knife up your penis and turned it around?

FRANK: I think I'd notice that.

SUE: I'm sure you would. And you don't gotta go to the bathroom a whole lot more than normal?

FRANK: No, I don't go to the bathroom more often than anybody else.

SUE: I'm sorry, I have no idea. Now, is it pleasurable?

FRANK: Not to the degree that you'd like . . .

SUE: Well, guys don't have cubicles, if you're standing in front of the urinal and you get that oh, oh, OH feeling . . .

FRANK: No, nothing like that. It's probably four percent of what you'd usually feel.

SUE: Gives you a silly grin afterwards.

FRANK: More of a stupid grin.

SUE: Frank, I really don't know. You've stumped me.

FRANK: Well, it happens most often after I ride my motorcycle. If I've driven the motorcycle for an hour or so, that's when it happens most.

SUE: They know that the vibrations from a motorcycle are stimulating to males.

FRANK: The same sort of thing — but a full-blown orgasm — happens when I do a lot of abdominal exercises, when I almost overdo it — crunches, sit-ups, that sort of thing.

SUE: It's a great incentive to exercise, I guess.

FRANK: (laughs)

SUE: I've heard of this happening to women. I've heard women at the Y say the exact same thing, that with certain exercises they'll have an orgasm. So if it works for you … you're not embarrassed … but what if you're wearing spandex? Does it get all bent out of shape?

FRANK: I exercise at home so that's not a problem. So, I don't have to worry about this though?

SUE: No, look at it this way — by exercising and masturbating at the same time, you're just multi-tasking. Enjoy!

> **One in ten thousand men have their first heart attack while having sex; only one in one million have a repeat attack during sex.**

Another trend we've noticed since the show began is the growing fascination with anal intercourse. In the first two seasons, questions about "bum sex," as Sue puts it, were few and far between, and usually from gay males. Now it's a common question, often from a woman who is feeling pressured by her boyfriend to try it. Anal intercourse avoids a potential pregnancy, it's true, but presents a whole panoply of other problems, not the least of which is pain. Then there's possible rectal bleeding, anal fissures, sexually transmitted diseases, and an ever-slackening sphincter. As Sue has pointed out many times, God gave us a sphincter so we could eat pork and beans.

When You Gotta Go . . .

SUE: Hey, we've got Janice from Burnaby waiting on the line. Hi Janice.

JANICE: Hi Sue. I have a friend who's been in a long-term relationship with a guy. She told me that they are very compatible sexually. He prefers anal sex and that's not a problem for her, but what he does after is a bit strange to me. He comes that way and then he will urinate in her.

SUE: (she flinches) In her rectum?

JANICE: Yes . . . and of course there's a reaction after . . .

SUE: I would imagine so. From a medical perspective, this is not dangerous. Urine is sterile; your bowel is not sterile — your bowel is loaded with caca and bacteria, but urine is sterile so if he urinates in her rectum, it acts very much like an enema.

JANICE: That's what I figured.

SUE: She'd get it all back in about 20 minutes. And how does she feel about that?

JANICE: It doesn't seem to bother her or else she wouldn't have told me about it.

SUE: If it doesn't bother her then okay, that's fine. Medically she's fine. I mean it's not an everyday common practice but it is okay. You know what I'm wondering? How can he urinate right after he ejaculates?

Most males have a little valve in the urethra that shuts off so that, when sperm come up from the testicles and mix with seminal fluid, this valve cuts off so that the ejaculate doesn't go up into his bladder. Well, it takes a few seconds for guys to urinate as they have to wait for that valve to open up.

JANICE: I don't know.

SUE: Well, ask her about that. If there's a time lag, then he's normal.

JANICE: Good, he's normal. Like I say, they do have a compatible sexual relationship, but I was concerned about that because it's so odd.

SUE: I've certainly heard about it before and it's not something that's that unusual. Luckily she has a good friend like you to talk to about this.

JANICE: Yeah, and I can talk to you and I'm glad I asked. Thank you Sue.

> The custom of denoting a brothel with
> a red lantern was established by law in
> Avignon, France in 1234.

Over the centuries, men have proven to be proficient at aiming crossbows and Cruise missiles, but we seem to be inept when it comes to aiming a penis. The average penis, generally smaller than a Cruise missile, should be easy to control but many callers have claimed otherwise.

Better Than a Sharp Stick

SUE: And from Medicine Hat, we've got Wendy on the line. Hi Wendy.

WENDY: Hi Sue. I just have a safety question. My boyfriend loves oral sex and so do I, but last week we were in the 69 position and he accidentally poked me in the eye with his penis. (Sue chuckles.) Now it's irritated and I'm just worried there could be an infection.

SUE: Is there any possibility that he could have gonorrhoea?

WENDY: I don't know. He has had a lot of girlfriends and he's been quite promiscuous in the past, so it's a possibility.

SUE: Is there any discharge?

WENDY: Not that I've noticed. From my eye or from his penis? (They both start laughing.)

SUE: No, from your eye.

WENDY: From my eye, not a lot, but it's been watering pretty constantly.

SUE: I'm just wondering if you're just too conscious of it. I'm not sure, but if there's any discharge, I would hightail it down to the doctor pretty quickly. Gonorrhoea is the one I would worry about the most, although if he had herpes on his penis then there's a possibility that the herpes virus could get into your eye. This is not likely, but if you're not sure, I would just go to the doctor and get it checked out.

WENDY: Okay, thank you.

SUE: And, in future, you might want to wear a diving mask to bed.

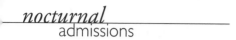

I Can't Hear You . . . Part Two

SUE: We've got Emily on the line from Moncton. You've got a question?

EMILY: I feel very uncomfortable talking about this, but, before we have sexual intercourse, my boyfriend likes to stick his penis in my ear.

SUE: In your ear!

EMILY: Yes. I don't know why, but this somehow turns him on. It just makes me feel really weird and I don't know how to tell him because, if we don't do this, he doesn't want to have sex.

SUE: Okay, that sounds a little bit like a fetish. It almost sounds as though this is something that he's fantasized about for years and he can't get aroused if he doesn't put his penis in your ear. Now, how far in your ear can you put a penis? Not very far, I should think!

EMILY: No, well not really.

SUE: I can't understand what's the thrill there. I can understand blowing in your ear, sucking your ear, yeah — but sticking his penis in your ear does sound a little bit like a fetish. My concern is that I want you to look five years down the road and, are you still going to be with this guy?

EMILY: I don't know.

SUE: Because then, if you don't know and you're not committed to this relationship, say, "You know what? I'm sorry but as far as I'm concerned, sticking your penis in my ear is not part of my sexual arousal. In fact, it turns me right off, and I don't want to have sex at all. So, either you give up the penis in the ear bit or we give up sex 'cause I'm just not interested in that. I don't want to do it; it just turns me off." Be very honest, very up-front and talk about it to try to find out where this came from. But, you know what, it doesn't much matter where it came from because, as long as he insists that's what he wants to do, then that's his fetish. It's not your fetish and therefore, hey, I'm sorry but it's not going to work.

EMILY: You know what, you're right Sue. Thanks.

> In the U.S., one teenager becomes pregnant every 20 seconds.

Let's face it, the penis is not the only body part that men have trouble with. "Dangly bits" just seem to be ripe for all manner of mishap . . .

Just Called to Brag

SUE: Now we've got Josh on the phone. Hi Josh.

JOSH: I have enormously large testicles. I was wondering if there is something wrong?

SUE: Are they painful?

JOSH: No.

SUE: Can you still walk?

JOSH: Yes.

SUE: You're fine.

Bic's Pickle

SUE: And from Edmonton, we've got Jim calling. Hi Jim.

JIM: Hi Sue. I did something tonight for my girlfriend. I shaved myself and I kinda cut myself very badly.

SUE: (Mouth open) Oh, really!

JIM: Yeah, and it was kinda hard to stop it from bleeding, but I did stop it from bleeding and I'm kinda wondering what I should do?

SUE: It's in the pubic hair area?

JIM: Down on the bottom of the shaft.

SUE: Man, you can't even put a Band-Aid there. Okay, get some of that antibiotic cream. Go to the drugstore. Got an all-night drugstore?

JIM: I did put some antibiotic cream on it.

SUE: Okay, that'll do it. Fine. And now, no sex. Like no sex.

JIM: How long?

SUE: Well, until it's healed up completely, closed over, no scars, and no scab. You can get an infection. You can get a nasty infection. *You don't want it.* You could get a lovely abscess there. So, you know, "Not tonight dear. I've got a sore." And next time you shave yourself, be gentle. Okay. And please do your girlfriend a favour . . . don't try shaving her. . . . Oh gee.

Nut Cracker

SUE: Looks like we have Megan from Timmins on the line. Hi Megan. What's your question?

MEGAN: My husband does this weird thing with his penis, where he'll push it down and it cracks.

SUE: Yeah, I've heard that before too and it's called fractured penis.

It sounds like you're pulling your knuckles, that popping sound.

MEGAN: Yeah. Is it bad for him?

SUE: I have never heard of any real negatives from it. Now, is it pleasurable? Is it, "Hey, look what I can do?" Or does it feel good to do it?

MEGAN: Well, I just know that he likes doing it because he's never heard about anyone else who can do it.

SUE: So, he does it because nobody else can do it. Something he can do better. Then I think you should pretend that you're very, very impressed. Just look at him and say, "Wow, I wish I could do that! I wish I had a toy like that." Never mind — you've got vaginal farts, they can't do that. (They laugh.) So, he can crack his penis and you can vaginal fart.

MEGAN: Is it bad for him?

SUE: It's not good, it's not bad. It won't do him damage. It's like cracking your knuckles even though people told you you might get arthritis.

MEGAN: Can he get arthritis from that?

SUE: No, no, because the penis has no bone. He's fine. You two are going to make a great pair, popping and farting in bed. Glad I'm not in the next room. Ha!

Too Dumb to Fuck

SUE: Looks like we've got Chuck from North Bay on the line. Hi Chuck.

CHUCK: Hi Sue. Usually when I'm out with my friends I drink a little too much. Like, I can't usually get it up sometimes.

SUE: Yeah, two drinks and you can do anything, three drinks and you can't do nothing. So what's the clue here?

CHUCK: That I'm drinking too much? But is there any way to still get it up and still drink lots with my buddies?

SUE: (incredulous) *Nooo.* You see, when you drink a lot of alcohol, you reduce the sensations, you know that. You know when you imbibe, you've been drinking too much, you're stumbling, your co-ordination is off, you know that you don't feel things as much, you're numb. And your penis is numb, too, so there's no stimulation getting through from the brain to the penis. So, what you gotta do is stop after two drinks. If you wanna have sex, you say, "I'm sorry. I've got better plans for tonight. I'm not drinking," and that's it.

CHUCK: Oh, okay.

SUE: And if you drink more than three, you just say, "Goodnight dear, that's it, game over, can't do nothing." Sorry Chuck. Drinks and dinks do not mix.

♀♂

Whereas men have their gender peculiarities, women are not immune to some odd sexual notions of their own. I shouldn't say "odd" — let's say "different."

Depends . . .

SUE: Now we've got Walter on the line from Regina.

WALTER: Hi Sue. My girlfriend enjoys being treated like an infant.

SUE: Oh, she wants to be the baby. She wants the rattle and the soother, and she wants the diapers. Now does she like to have you change her diapers?

WALTER: Well, yeah, and she wants me to stimulate her by rubbing her down there while I do it.

SUE: This is a form of fetish and it is called "infantilism."

WALTER: Is this a normal thing to carry this out?

SUE: If it's pleasurable for her and acceptable to you, then it's normal. If you're comfortable with it, if you get sexually aroused and you think it's fun, and if you can get into that role playing, then there's nothing wrong with it.

WALTER: Okay.

SUE: Now sometimes it goes even further than that. Sometimes the people who are involved in infantilism also like to urinate in the diaper and also have a bowel movement in the diaper. The turn-on for them is to have somebody change the diaper, somebody to clean up.

WALTER: That's disgusting.

SUE: Okay, Walter, you seem very clear on that. You have to set the limits on what you feel comfortable with, and then carry on from there.

WALTER: Okay.

SUE: If it's really bothering you, then you'd better talk with her about it. It may be time to throw the baby out with the bath-water.

50% of women have one breast that is larger than the other.

No Shit

SUE: From Kelowna, we've got Jim on the line. Got a problem, Jim?

JIM: My girlfriend says I'm not satisfying her sexually, and I'm worried that she's going to leave me. One alternative method she's brought up is defecating on her breasts.

SUE: (shocked) Well, that's quite a leap from not satisfying her sexually to defecating on her breasts. That tells me that she has flipped into this fantasy about scat — that's what it's called when you're into defecation with sex.

JIM: Yeah, she even brings up urinating too.

SUE: And how do you feel about that?

JIM: Well, I'm just not entirely comfortable. I'd like to leave that in the washroom. Sometimes she wants me to rub it on her and stuff. I just don't understand it.

SUE: Now, you've got to decide how you feel about being involved in sex with faeces and with urine. That's gotta be your decision. And if you decide that this is caca, this is poo-poo, and you're not going there, you just explain it to her and say, "For me, this is gross. It's not something I'm interested in, not something I even want to try." You make the call, it's your decision. Don't let anybody talk you into doing things that you don't want to do, that you're uncomfortable with, or that you regard as simply abnormal or unacceptable. She'll just have to find another way to be satisfied.

There's one type of call we occasionally receive that you'll never hear on air — people who have sex with their dogs. It's uncommon, but we do get a few. I remember Sue telling us about a letter she had received from a woman who had photos of her

German shepherd and shots of it having intercourse with her. Apparently, the dog was wearing little booties so it wouldn't scratch her back.

I also remember a gay friend of mine having a date with a guy who invited him back to his place. He had a lovely Doberman at home who was particularly friendly. After making out on the couch for a while, the guy invited my friend into the bedroom. They disrobed, and as they climbed into bed, he said, "You don't mind if the dog joins us, do you?" Well, that was it. My friend bolted with his tail between his legs, as it were. I have a terrible feeling that bestiality is more common than we think. Of course, it *is* illegal and we strongly recommend that you not look for a date at the local pound.

Animal Love

SUE: And now we've got Brenda on the line from Toronto. Hi Brenda.

BRENDA: I have this weird problem, not really me, but my boyfriend. He's got this fetish where he likes to role play when we have sex. But the problem is he likes to act like animals. Have you ever seen documentaries of animals mating?

SUE: Yeesssss . . .

BRENDA: He wants us to act like wild animals who have wild sex drives. He wants me to act like different animals — like occasionally we'll do it like giraffes, and elephants, and lions. I feel really uncomfortable, but I don't want to tell him because I went along with him for a while.

SUE: You're talking about rear entry?

BRENDA: Yes, rear entry and other positions, but just pretending we're like animals. I just find it uncomfortable.

SUE: Does he want to do this all the time, every time?

BRENDA: Yeah. Is there something I can do to boost our sex lives? Is there something I'm doing wrong, or is this just him?

SUE: No, I think it's probably him. I don't know that it's a problem, it's just something he finds very exciting, watching animals mating. He gets turned on. There are lots of books around for spicing up your sex life, so you could pick up one of those.

BRENDA: Have you ever heard of this before?

SUE: No, I haven't, but it wouldn't be something that would really upset me. I'm trying to think of different animals and how they mate. I'm thinking of snakes.

BRENDA: Oh, he watches them all and he tapes the shows and he shows them to me and says this is how I want it done. And I say okay.... But I'm not an elephant and I'm not a tiger ...

SUE: Obviously, you're uncomfortable with this. You've gotta tell him that you're having trouble dealing with this. You've given it a fair trial, goodness knows. You've done it, you've tried it, and it doesn't do a thing for you.

BRENDA: And it's exhausting too.

SUE: Well, unless you're a tree sloth. No, you've gotta say, "This is something that doesn't appeal to me at all, so, we've got to find some other way of doing this because it's just not working out." But do it now, before it goes much further, because he doesn't know how you feel.

BRENDA: Yeah, I've been faking it, faking like an animal.

SUE: Well, I think it's time to be honest.

BRENDA: Okay, thanks, appreciate it.

Animals have to deal with technological aggravation — such as documentary filmmakers spying on them while they're having sex — just as humans do. There was an infamous, behind-the-scenes technical failure on the *Sunday Night Sex Show* when the entire studio crew got trapped in the elevator at SkyDome. Unfortunately, no one in the Control Room knew they were absent until five minutes to air. Then we panicked. A repeat program was in the works but, at one minute to air, the gang came running down the hall and leapt into position. The show went on with viewers none the wiser. Some of our callers have had their own technological challenges . . .

Brace Yourself

SUE: And we've got Brian on the line from Whitehorse. Hi Brian. Got a question?

BRIAN: When my girlfriend gives me oral sex, she has braces and sometimes it's uncomfortable. Do you have any pointers?

SUE: (She winces) Oh, braces. Ouch, they hurt — all metal? Around every tooth? How about if you wear a condom?

BRIAN: We've tried it and it doesn't help.

SUE: What, you end up with a tattered condom?

BRIAN: Yes.

SUE: Brian, I have no idea what you can do. She's going to have to perform oral sex with her lips over her teeth. That's the only way she can do it. I'm sorry!

BRIAN: Guess she's going to need bigger lips then.

SUE: Or you need a smaller penis. (He laughs.) Sorry, Brian, but until those braces come off, there's nothing you can do.

A Little Dab'll Do Ya

SUE: Now we've got James on the line from Thunder Bay. Hi James. Got a question?

JAMES: It's kind of embarrassing, but it's a common problem, I think. I'm a gay male in a relationship, and I want to know if there's a trick or a product you can use to get cum out of your hair? Like, you go into the shower afterwards and it bakes into it.

SUE: (giggles) Oh. Is there a trick or a product to get ejaculate out of your hair? It's gotta be better than hair spray. I can't think of anything that's going to work better than soap and water. You may have to wash your hair twice, give it two shampoos, and then brush it later to get the — pardon the expression — get the "stiffness" out.

JAMES: Yeah, well, it's almost like having gum in your hair. Is there something you can use? Someone should invent that!

SUE: James, I've been in this business for over 20 years and I've never heard this problem before. Normally shampoo bottles just list qualities like taming dandruff or dry scalp, but I've never seen one that says, "Guaranteed to Remove Cum." So I think you're going to have to experiment with different shampoos, some are stronger than others, just experiment and find one that works. I mean, James, when you have sex and some of his ejaculate gets on your pubic hair, does it stay there forever and ever, amen?

JAMES: No, but what if you're performing oral sex and it gets in your hair? Even when you go in the shower right away hoping to get it out — I don't know what that stuff's made of, but it bakes into your hair like melted plastic.

SUE: Best I can suggest, James. Or else, just aim it away from you. You're holding his penis — point it at *him*.

JAMES: I tried that but he shoots a lot.

SUE: Honey, have you ever held a hose and watered the garden? Well, you probably didn't spray yourself in the head, and he probably doesn't shoot more than that. You can do it!

JAMES: I'll try it. Thanks Sue.

♀♂

Some calls make us giggle, just as they do to viewers, but most questions are fairly routine. We've all become amateur "sexperts" after six seasons. A couple of times, though, we've had calls that were so upsetting that people in the Control Room began to cry. Such a call is very, very difficult to work through. The only way to get through it is to separate yourself from what's happening, and weep in the commercial break. This was one of those calls . . .

SUE: We've got Connor on the line from St. John's. Hi Connor.

CONNOR: I just found out about a week ago that I'm HIV positive. I've been seeing this girl for a few months, and I don't know how to break it to her.

SUE: That's really tough. Now, when you were diagnosed, did the doctor or clinic spend some time talking to you about your relationship with your partner?

CONNOR: That's not the only problem. I've also had sexual relationships with two other girls.

SUE: Is there a possibility you might have infected them?

CONNOR: I didn't use protection at all.

SUE: Do you know approximately when you contracted the disease?

CONNOR: I don't know.

SUE: Well, you're going to have to tell them.

CONNOR: I just feel like running away.

SUE: I know. But that's unfair because they will be totally unsuspecting. And we know that, particularly for females, early diagnosis and initiating treatment really early on is really beneficial.

CONNOR: I heard about some sort of antibiotic ...

SUE: There is a treatment, but that has to be initiated very early on.

CONNOR: It's been more than a week.

SUE: You know what. First, I would definitely tell them. And then they can go to their doctor or an HIV clinic and ask about this prophylactic treatment. They use it mainly for doctors and nurses who may have got needle injuries.

CONNOR: I'm not a needle user.

SUE: So you know you got it from sex. Were you ever involved in a same sex relationship?

CONNOR: No.

SUE: So, you got infected from a female. Which is kind of unusual. So, one of these females is infected already and doesn't know it. So, you have an obligation to tell all of them.

CONNOR: I have to tell them.

SUE: (pleading) Yeah, you do. Honey, if you were intimate enough to have sex with them ...

CONNOR: These were one-night stands.

SUE: I know, but that's still intimacy. It's not long-term intimacy or loving intimacy, but it was still intimacy.

CONNOR: I can't find one of the two girls.

SUE: You don't know any of her friends?

CONNOR: I met her at a bar.

SUE: Now, how are we going to word this? Because, obviously, you're having trouble articulating the fact that you are infected. What do you want to say to them?

CONNOR: I don't know. I just want to jump off a bridge and just . . .

SUE: Oh, okay, no, don't do that.

CONNOR: I don't know what to do, Sue.

SUE: Will you go back to the HIV clinic and get some counselling?

CONNOR: I don't know what to do . . .

SUE: You've got to get back to that clinic right away, because obviously this is very upsetting for you. And it's much, much more than you worrying about the girls. I realize that's a component of it (Connor starts crying), so will you go back to counselling? I have a phone number for you, can you take down this number? (She gives number.) Now, don't hang up, stay on the phone. After we are finished, our call screener will give you that number in case you didn't have a pencil handy. Have you got a support system at all? Anybody close enough you can talk to?

CONNOR: I phoned my mom and told her.

SUE: Does she live in the same area?

CONNOR: (sobbing) No.

SUE: Can you get home to her?

CONNOR: No.

SUE: Then you have to get to the AIDS Committee. I know them in your city and they are wonderful. They may not be open Sunday night. Can you hang in until tomorrow?

CONNOR: I don't know . . .

SUE: You can, you can. Now, if you're feeling really desperate, would you go to Emergency?

CONNOR: What can they do?

SUE: They can listen to you, and talk to you and talk about the fact that this is not the end of your life, believe me. They'll help you come to terms with the fact that, yes, you are infected, how are we going to handle this and find some way of living with it. Would you do that tonight?

CONNOR: I'll phone the number you've given me.

SUE: We'll check during the break to see if that number is on tonight. Don't go away. Stay there. . . . I'm sorry. Hang on, honey.

Connor didn't hang on — he hung up. We called the AIDS Committee right away to let them know what had happened. The next day, Sue called every hospital listed for that city, looking for Connor. She couldn't find him, although it's unlikely that Emergency Rooms would have revealed that personal information anyway. WTN was flooded with calls from viewers who had watched the show, offering their sympathy and support. We wondered how many other people had been through the same terrible, emotional ordeal he was going through. Connor never called back. Connor, if you're reading this, please let us know how you are. Hanging on, we hope and pray.

The Agony Aunt

The *Sunday Night Sex Show* is part of a media tradition that stretches back over 300 years — the "Agony Aunt." An "Agony Aunt" is the generic term for an advice columnist. The first one appeared in England in 1691, published by Londoner John Dunton. Dunton was having an affair, and felt his own need for unbiased, outside advice. By 1693, his popular publication had evolved into *The Ladies' Mercury*. In her paper, "An Anatomy of Advice," Frances Bartlett writes, "Within its pages, he promised, were answers to 'all the most nice and curious questions concerning love, marriage behaviour, dress and humour of the female sex, whether virgins, wives or widows.'" She also notes that the letters chosen for publication were chosen with male readers in mind, and were sufficiently bawdy to engage the casual reader. Sound familiar?

Perils of the Pleasure Chest

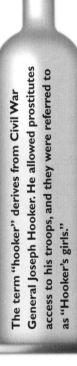

The term "hooker" derives from Civil War General Joseph Hooker. He allowed prostitutes access to his troops, and they were referred to as "Hooker's girls."

Without question, the most popular segment of the *Sunday Night Sex Show* is the "Pleasure Chest." It's the segment people wait up for or switch the channel to see. We try to place it at the end of the 11:00 p.m. news in Ontario because, really, it's a public service. We'd rather viewers fell asleep dreaming about the "Deep Penetrating Dong" than the "Deep, Penetrating Deficit."

Sue used to find the toys herself, rounding them up at Aren't We Naughty, her local sex shop. When she turned up with "The Juicer," we thought maybe it was time to send somebody else. Now Corey Silverberg, who co-owns a sex store called Come As You Are, is our sex toy sleuth. He provides most of the items for the "Pleasure Chest" — along with prices and his professional comments. Other items are sent to the show by manufacturers hoping for a good review, plus Sue still drags in the odd toy she finds

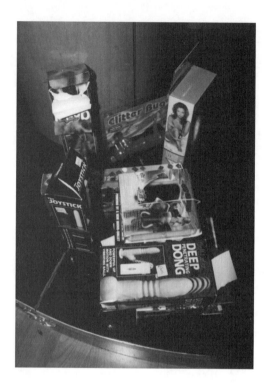

*"Crew bonus" piling
up in preparation for
the Sex Toy Scramble.*

in her travels — "erotic souvenirs," as it were. No matter what she says about a device, sex shops from coast to coast are besieged with customers looking for the item the next day. In fact, stores have asked us for advance warning so they can stock up on the toy we'll be showing. Needless to say, the folks at Duracell are big fans of our show.

When it's anatomically possible, someone on the crew risks their genitalia to test a product and send a report back from the "front." Over the last few years, there's been some high-lights and a lot of low-lights . . .

The Juicer

Who could forget "The Juicer"? Sue decided she would do a segment on butt plugs, a topic not regularly featured on *Oprah*. A butt plug, for the uninitiated (and that's most of us), is a rubber or latex phallus of varying size that one places in the anus and leaves there for an extended period of time. Placed there, a butt plug can provide mild stimulation throughout the day as well as keep your rectum loose for potential anal intercourse later. I always think they should build a whistle into them. It'd be great for party tricks.

Generally, a butt plug is harmless. It's a conical shape, with a narrow head that widens out into a bulbous middle, and then has a narrow base with a wide flange on its bottom so it won't completely disappear into, well, *your* bottom. Picture a spade from a deck of cards and you'll know what a butt plug looks like. It doesn't vibrate and has no motor. It just sits there, acting, literally, as a plug held in place by the sphincter muscle. Butt plugs usually range in length from three to five inches, and are only a couple of inches wide at their widest point. Anyway, that's what we thought, until Sue found "The Juicer."

As I recall, "The Juicer" looked exactly like its namesake, a grapefruit juicer, with a much higher point and broader base. It was made of hard latex. Unlike most butt plugs, it didn't narrow down at the base. It got distressingly wide and stayed wide. Unless there were some butt-hole surfing elephants watching, I don't think there was a single viewer who didn't shriek when Sue held it up. Everyone in the Control Room did. You could have plugged the leak in the Titanic with this baby.

The funny thing was my friend Jordan. He'd been watching the news and innocently flipped over just in time to see

Sue hold up "The Juicer." He claims that he regained con-
sciousness *before* the medics arrived.

[Note from the crew: *Nobody* tried "The Juicer," except for
making breakfast.]

Although anal stimulation can be extremely pleasurable, there
are many items (besides "The Juicer") that one should avoid
inserting in one's ass. The Internet, that vast storehouse of
questionable knowledge, offers many Web sites that describe
items removed from anal canals in hospital Emergency
Rooms. The patient is invariably male and always has the same
story: he accidentally "fell" on it. Right. Here's what some
guys have "fallen" on:

- a can of "Impulse Body Spray"
- Coke bottles
- lightbulbs
- axe handles
- broom handles (the most common mishap)
- paintbrushes
- hammer handles
- apples
- carrots
- plantains
- cucumbers (of course)
- a turnip
- a mortar pestle
- knife sharpeners
- an ice pick (youch!)
- spatulas
- a tin cup
- candles
- flashlights (guess they forgot to light the candles)
- pens
- screwdrivers
- toothbrushes
- toothbrush holders
- baseballs
- baseball bats
- tennis balls
- tennis racket handles
- baby powder cans
- a snuff box
- cattle horns

- frozen pig's tail (at least they got the location right)
- large stones
- whip handles
- cans of motor oil
- a toolbox

Obviously guys have a poor sense of balance, and they should always exercise extreme caution when walking naked near any lubricated objects.

The Blowup Doll

Sue rarely loses a battle, but she lost this one.

Next to dildos — which go back thousands of years — blowup dolls are one of the oldest sex toys around. Many people, Sue included, regard them as a joke and not as a serious erotic toy. Nonetheless, she decided to cover them in the "Pleasure Chest" and to have two fully-clothed blowup dolls, male and female, sitting with her on the set. In December 1999, she faxed this script to Julie:

"Meet my date, Studleigh. Studleigh doesn't have much going for him. His hair is a disaster, he is under five feet tall, his skin is cold and clammy, he smells like plastic, and his penis comes off. Not my idea of a hot date.

"Then, there's Stella, Studleigh's girlfriend. She is something else. Big mouth, bed head hair, and a stiff, cold plastic body. Stella comes equipped with a removable one-piece Cyber Skin vagina and rectum. At $162 plus taxes, Stella is not cheap.

"Don't try to fill these dolls with helium; you'll have trouble getting them off the ceiling. And don't bite — they'll let you down . . . badly.

"From what I hear, Stella and Studleigh are primarily gag gifts you give to someone for their 50th birthday. Then they get stored on the top shelf of a cupboard until the grandchildren find them.

"There's also a Cyber Skin doll which, for US$5,000, is made to order and comes in a box shaped like a casket. Try explaining that to your wife."

Some people, on the other hand, do not see the humour in blowup dolls at all. They are, in fact, deeply offended by them. One such person is Julie Smith.

"Sue, we are not doing blowup dolls," says Julie in the pre-show meeting. It's not unusual for Julie to say "No" and then come around, but this time she looks determined.

"Why not?" Sue protests. "They're absolutely hilarious and one of the oldest sex toys around."

"Sue, they're offensive. They objectify women."

"Well, don't vibrators objectify men?"

"That's different. Vibrators just represent one body part, not a whole body. A blowup doll with its open mouth and open vagina is just plain sick. They give me the creeps."

Sue's not buying this argument, sensing a personal bias behind it. "The purpose of the 'Pleasure Chest' is to show consumers what's out there. They've all seen blowup dolls, Julie. They're even used in movies for gags. I'm just going to trash them anyway."

"Personally, I find them extremely offensive, but I'll ask the ladies at the office and see what other people think. Then, we'll see." Julie shuts down the discussion.

The rest of the evening was a bit tense, with both ladies giving the topic a wide berth.

Producing a television show is not a science. It is completely reliant on gut instinct. As the producer, Julie has to go by what feels right to her. That's her job. A good producer goes by her or his gut, and — if they have a good one — the show gets good ratings. If they don't, the show gets cancelled. They're not always right (see _Ralph Benmurgui_) but, ultimately, someone on the show has to make a final decision on content.

Unfortunately, producers, being only human, suffer from the same idiosyncrasies we all suffer from. Sometimes they have a niggling little irrational thing that really bugs them. I worked on the _Dini_ show with an outside consultant for a while, a person whom I grew to love and admire. But even this programming genius had a pet bugaboo — the word "fart." No one was allowed to say the word on _Dini_, neither host nor guest. They could say "shit" and "piss me off," but nary a "fart" was heard. Our consultant thought the word was very offensive and should never be broadcast.

Having conducted an office survey, Julie returned the following week to report that her staff was as offended as she was. "Well, Sue, the ladies in the office totally agree with me. We won't be doing blowup dolls on the _Sunday Night Sex Show_." Sue merely snorted her annoyance.

Neither Studleigh nor Stella have made an appearance yet, and it's unlikely that they ever will. That didn't stop us from teasing Julie, however.

Shortly after this incident, Julie was snowed in while on a business trip to Winnipeg. She couldn't make it back for the show, which left me in charge. When she called just before airtime from the Fort Garry Hotel to see how things were shaping up, I reassured her.

"No problem, Julie, we're doing an entire hour on blowup dolls — from an S&M gay bar. You'll love it!" I think I heard the bar fridge open.

The Vacuum Pump

Before Viagra appeared on the scene, the vacuum pump was one of the best methods available for coaxing a workable erection out of an indifferent penis. It's still the safest method of choice for those with high blood pressure or a heart condition.

It works on a simple principle: a penis expands inside a vacuum. The device is fairly ungainly. It consists of a long, clear Plexiglas tube (sort of like a Patty Stacker, but not as wide); a pump mechanism that screws on to the top of the tube to make an airtight seal; a hose ending in a hand-operated, rubber vacuum bulb that gets squeezed to draw the air out; a valve to release the vacuum; and a cock-ring that fits around the open end of the tube.

You place the device tightly over the penis and pump the air out with the vacuum bulb. As a vacuum forms inside, blood is naturally drawn into the penis, creating an erection. Then, you open the valve to release the vacuum, withdraw the pump, and slip the cock-ring over the base of the penis to keep the blood inside. The result? It's not hard enough to strike matches on, but it's a serviceable erection.

The pump Sue received was a legitimate medical device that came with a carrying case and an instructional videotape. Some unscrupulous manufacturers try to pass off cheap vacuum pumps as a device to increase penis size. Yes, a penis does get bigger in a vacuum — which will add a certain allure to space travel — but, for a permanent increase, you'd have better luck tying a rope around your dick, hooking it to the back of a pick-up truck, and telling Jeb to drive away fast. We don't recommend this method.

When the pump was delivered to Sue's condo, she was so excited that she didn't really study the instructions as well as she should have. In fact, she completely missed the part about the release valve. She managed to assemble it (no small feat), stretched the lubricated cock-ring over the open end, and tried the pump on the palm of her hand. This wasn't working. She needed a larger area of flesh. Her stomach seemed like an obvious choice.

Holding the base flat against her abdomen, she pumped away. A dome of fat, resembling those unnaturally slow bubbles that percolate in molten lava, rose up into the tube. Soon she had a penis-sized bubble of blubber sucked in. Judging the demonstration a success, she tried to pull the device off. It wouldn't budge. She pulled harder. It refused to let go. Starting to panic, she tugged, yanked, and spun around in circles as the flesh inside started to turn a bright shade of scarlet. Sue was getting the biggest hickey she'd ever had in her life. Finally, she spied the release valve and smacked it. As the tube popped off, the cock-ring slipped onto the bottom of the slab of flab, and suddenly, she had an extra appendage poking out of her tummy. "Pinch an inch" started to seem like a enviable goal. Struggling with the cock-ring and quite thoroughly bruising herself in the process, Sue ultimately managed to free herself from the diabolical flesh-eating machine.

So, it was with a certain amount of trepidation that she pulled the vacuum pump out of the "Pleasure Chest" on air.

Things started off fine. She greased up the cock-ring and

stretched it over one end of the tube. In hindsight, this was the part of the procedure she should have done *last*. Now her hands were slippery. As she tried to attach the pump mechanism on the other end, it shot away from her and went sailing across the studio, landing off-camera with a hollow, plastic thud. Sue started giggling while Germain ran after the piece. Next thing we saw was a black hand come up from behind the desk, offering her the wayward apparatus. She grabbed it, and gamely carried on with her Very Important Demo. It was, after all, live television. Flustered, she tried to jam the pump into position. This proved to be an excellent example of the scientific principle of action/reaction as the entire device launched like a missile from her desktop, crashing in several pieces on the studio floor.

By this time, Sue had completely lost it. She collapsed in laughter, gasping and choking, and confessed the whole, sorry, hickey incident. The faithful Germain retrieved the scattered bits and Sue did, eventually, manage to get the thing assembled. But seeing the vacuum pump in action was an anti-climax, as it were. In this case, the foreplay was all the fun.

Sue's Rant

Nothing gets Sue going like a ridiculously expensive sex toy. As far as she's concerned, sex shouldn't cost any more than one condom. In January 2000, she started the millennium with this pecuniary rant about the very pricey "G-Spot Tango":

"I took one look at the price tag on the 'G-Spot Tango' at $109.99 plus taxes, and I decided it had better be bloody good for that price.

"Maybe I have been watching too much _ER_, but it looks like an endotracheal tube with a defibrillator to me. If somebody came at me with this thing, I'd think I was dead!

"'G-Spot Tango' is a fuchsia vibrator with a rotating head and a control panel that looks like the cockpit of an airplane. This extension cord connects the vibrating suction 'kisser' with its vibrating pistolettes. It does everything but wash the windows.

"Now, guys can use it too, although it is a bit large for anal stimulation, but the 'kisser' could be used to stimulate the testicles and penis. It takes three AA batteries.

"But, you know what? If you have 10 fingers and a tongue, you can do the same thing and save yourself about 130 bucks. Plus, you won't have to hide this from the kids."

I'll bet they still sold thousands of them the next day.

The Chin Dong

It sounded like a Szechuan appetizer, but when Sue pulls it out of her bag in the production meeting, it is a flesh-coloured, rubber dildo with straps. We are baffled.

"It's called a 'chin dong,'" she explains as she puts it on. A contoured cup in the base of the dildo deftly fits over her chin, and then the straps hook behind her head. The stiff phallus is now sticking straight out from her chin. As she talks, it waggles about obscenely.

"This is a great sex toy for paraplegics or quadriplegics," Sue continues. This is one of her pet projects, finding ways to give a sex life back to those who are disabled. "Anyone with limited head and neck movement can use this to satisfy their partner. They can perform oral sex on the clitoris and insert the dildo into the vagina at the same time."

As it flops around, we are all suppressing giggles — she is looking alarmingly like Brian Mulroney.

"Oh, I see," says Julie. "But you don't have to be disabled to use it. Anybody could use it."

"Absolutely. Oral sex would be great with this. I just hope I can get it to stay on on-air."

Julie looks alarmed but doesn't say anything. At least it's not a blowup doll.

So, there was Sue on national television with this six-inch, flesh-coloured dildo sticking out of her chin, earnestly explaining its merits as it flapped about in front of her, and behaving as if she was doing nothing more outrageous than delivering a weather report. She only stumbled when she caught a glimpse of herself on the studio monitor.

"There are times," she recalls, "when I say to myself, 'Susie, what are you doing? You look like a complete idiot!' That was one of those moments."

When Toys Go Bad — The Deep Penetrating Dong

I wish I could have seen the Customs Officer's face when these turned up at the border.

Customs Officer: "Have you got anything to declare?"

Truck Driver: "I've got four dozen 'Deep Penetrating Dongs.'"

Customs Officer: "Let me give you my home number."

The inventors of the "Deep Penetrating Dong" had noble aspirations. They set out to make a vibrator that didn't just vibrate — they wanted to create a spectacular device whose head actually goes up and down, simulating the thrusts of a real, honest-to-goodness penis. To a bunch of men, it must have sounded like a great idea. If they'd bothered to ask any woman, however, they would have discovered that most women achieve orgasm from clitoral, not vaginal, stimulation, and saved themselves a whole pile of work.

As I recall, there were several challenges in the design: it required two motors (one to vibrate, and one to drive a piston up and down); the piston required a lot of room, since there had to be sufficient length for the top of the stroke and the bottom of the stroke; the material that covered the thrusting portion had to be flexible, able to expand and contract; and the whole apparatus needed a big mother of a power-pack to drive both motors. The power-pack proved to be the toy's downfall.

The "Deep Penetrating Dong" turned out to be huge, big enough to make mares nervous. All parties declined to test it. We inserted the four C batteries before the show and turned it on to make sure it was working. It was. The round head thrust up and down, exactly as promised, albeit making the type of noise that would lead your neighbours to think you were drilling for oil in your bedroom. Then, we placed it in the "Pleasure Chest," and went about our business.

It stayed there throughout the first half of the show, building up a head of steam.

"Do you smell something burning?" Sue asked Derrick and Germain in the commercial break just before the "Pleasure Chest" segment. She reached for the chest and set it on her desk.

They sniffed. "No," they responded.

Back from the break, Sue started her spiel about big, stupid vibrators. She threw open the lid to the "Pleasure Chest," and — to our horror — smoke billowed out of the interior. The "Deep Penetrating Dong" was shorting out!

"*Oh my God,* it's on fire!" she exclaimed, waving the smoke away. "Talk about a hot date!"

In the Control Room, we quickly checked the box to see if there was any mention of "Fire Hazard" in the instructions.

She pulled it out of the chest and turned it on, which seemed to solve the problem. True to form, just like most guys, as soon as you get them thrusting they're way past smouldering. Sue wrapped up her bit, plopped the Dong back into the "Pleasure Chest," and had Germain remove it to a safe distance, somewhere near second base.

The last we heard, the "Deep Penetrating Dong" is packing ice cream at Ben & Jerry's.

Dishonourable Mentions

In our sixth season, we decided to do not only a list of the top 10 toys of the year, but also a list of the worst. We had plenty to choose from. Here's a brief recap of items lining the absolute bottom of the garbage pail:

"The Tongue" — This device made "The Juicer" look downright elegant. It looked exactly — and I do mean exactly — like one of those gross cow tongues you see hanging in the window of a Greek butcher shop. Battery-powered, the tip slowly moved up and down in a creepy simulation of a tongue licking. I'm getting queasy just telling you about it. Next.

"Grape-Scented Butt Plug" — Why?

"Clit-Critter" — Another jel vibrator, this one shaped like an elephant with tusks. Mostly offensive for its name.

"The Gerbil" — And you thought they couldn't get any lower than "The Tongue"? As you might suspect, it's a slender wand designed for anal stimulation that has the plastic equivalent of a gerbil on the end of it. Thank God they didn't use a raccoon.

Homemade Sex Toys

Sue, being eternally cheap, conjures up a batch of her own homemade sex toys each season. Frequently, these have all the erotic appeal of *The Antiques Roadshow*.

For example, she came up with a "Bubble-Wrap Dildo." She tore a strip of bubble-wrap out of the inside of a padded envelope, rolled it up, and stuffed it into a condom. Not only did it look silly, it barely had the rigidity required to penetrate a bowl of Jello. Bubble-wrap: great for shipping; not so good for receiving.

Then there was the "Homemade Blindfold," a chance to get a little taste of some mild bondage. She read in a book somewhere about taking a pair of swimming-goggles and painting them black. This would, of course, ruin the goggles for swimming. So, Sue being Sue, she simply put duct-tape over them so she could use them again. Very seductive, if you're married to Red Green.

Her "Nipple Jewellery" required more dexterity. It involved black elastic-thread doubled through a plastic bead so it could be tightened. Then she added a jingle bell from a Christmas ornament to it. Germain was the willing model as she tied the gewgaw to one of his nipples and made him wiggle his chest in a sexy manner. Ideal for keeping mice out of the bedroom.

Our favourite, though, was "The Homemade Vagina." With unabashed innocence, she had taken an old cat-food can; cut the top and bottom off it; fitted two, large work-socks into the interior to give the inside a tighter fit; and covered the socks with a plastic bag from No Frills, holding it in place with a heavy-duty rubber band that she had saved from a bunch of broccoli. When I cut to a close-up of her bargain-basement vagina, the guys in the studio and everyone in the Control Room burst out laughing. There, staring back at us from the green label on the original tin, was the happy face of a nice, big, fat pussy.

Best of the "Chest"

The truth of the matter is that most sex toys are over-priced, over-hyped pieces of junk. Their packaging promises far more than they can deliver. For instance, we've discovered that, as a rule, the term "Variable Speed" is a loose translation of Chinese for "ON" or "OFF." We've ascertained that the phrase, "Sold as a Novelty Item," means "Stick this in one of your holes." "Flexible" means "Slightly more malleable than concrete"; "Realistic" means "Doesn't feel like cork"; and "Reach New Heights of Orgasmic Delight" means "Almost as good as sitting on a bus."

Men buy far more sex toys than women. Subsequently, the packaging usually features a blissed-out blonde in her birthday

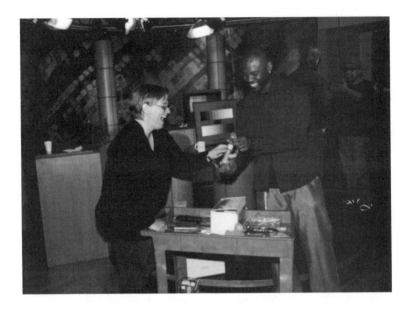

Frances and Germain share good vibrations.

suit, panting for more. Generally, her breasts contain six times more silicone than the toy in the box. When women buy toys, they tend to choose small, discreet vibrators, something suitable for clitoral stimulation. When guys buy a vibrator for their partner, they buy big, honking, penis-shaped monsters. As Sue has pointed out, Freud was wrong — it's men who suffer from penis envy, not women.

However, there are exceptions, and over the last few seasons, the *Sunday Night Sex Show* has offered its recap of the "Top Sex Toys of the Year" in its closing episode. These are toys that have been recommended by the crew and that actually work. We've rated them on a scale of one to four orgasms (****). So, if you want to spice up your sex life, here's a good place to start:

"Fukuoku" — This is Sue's all-time favourite sex toy, and she promoted it so much that we began to suspect that she had shares in the company. It's a tiny but powerful vibrator that is contoured to fit on the tip of a finger. It's powered by a tiny watch battery so there's no cord to get in the way. The "Fukuoku" is ideal for clitoral stimulation, which is what it's designed for, but it's just as sweet for stimulating the head of a penis or gently massaging the testicles.

It's pronounced *foo-ku-oh-ku*, but when it first turned up, we thought the name was *fuck you — okay you?* Duh. Talk about one-track minds. ****

"Cyber Cock" — This spectacular dildo not only looked like a real penis, it actually got warm when you held it. It's made of a new material that really *does* feel like skin — they're not lying. Sue's comments:

"'The Cyber Cock' feels so authentic — like real skin, not plastic — warm and human. The guys in my crew are pretty blasé about vibrators, but when they held this toy, they all agreed that this could make men redundant. Well, not quite. This does not snuggle, hug, kiss, or whisper sweet nothings in your ear — and it won't cut the lawn — but it will outlast most males. It's one of the best toys in my top 10 collection." ****

"Tickling Panties" — Sue said it all:
"We try to have members of the *Sunday Night Sex Show* crew 'test drive' each of our sex toys before I recommend them. It's a dirty job, but somebody's gotta do it. No problem with the 'Tickling Panties.' I was out of the running because these only

come in one size — not mine. Let me just tell you, the researcher spent an inordinate amount of time with a silly grin on her face. These special panties have a small, removable jelly-pad vibrator in the crotch and a hand-held, variable speed remote control, small and discreet. I think it's a brilliant device, but I'd suggest that the company make them in a large size, too. My concern is that you are driving to work, wearing these panties, and you have an orgasm. Puts a whole new meaning to 'rear-ender.' I'm not sure what your insurance company will think of your explanation. Just tell them, 'Sue says they work and I was just trying them out!'" ***

"The Wild Thing" — This is a passionate purple vibrator that has a long, narrow wand with a stiff, but flexible, shaft inside of it. It's perfect for anal stimulation because it's much smaller than a toolbox. Sue's review:
"For males who think that vibrators are just a 'girl thang,' we have 'The Wild Thang.' This is ideal for anal stimulation of the male's 'A' spot, and great for women as well. It is slender, making penetration painless, and is flexible but firm enough to allow for some gentle thrusting. The battery-powered bullet vibrator is quite powerful, and I'm told it stimulates an orgasm every time. You can't beat that." ****

"G-Spot Vibrator" — Over to Sue:
"Having trouble finding that elusive G-spot? Well, help is on the way. This vibrator is slightly curved about a third of the way down, so you can't miss. I'd suggest you experiment with this 'G-spot Vibrator' until you hit it right on. When you know where it's at, all you've got to do is guide your partner

— fingers or penis — hey, your G-spot isn't fussy! Getting there is half the fun. Do it on his side of the bed so you don't get the wet spot." ✳✳✳

"Deviant Liquid Body Paint" — We found this amazing product when we were shooting a story at a trade show, the "Everything to Do with Sex Show," held in Toronto in 2001. It's a paint kit of primary colours, and the paint is a thick, liquid latex that dries on the skin, and then peels off, keeping the exact shape it was painted over. So, you could paint yourself a skin-tight T-shirt, peel it off and put it back on again. Or you might want to try it on some other body parts. You could peel off some fascinating personal sculptures, guaranteed to offend the in-laws. Sue painted Germain's torso on air. We had to stop her there. ✳✳

"Jel-Lee 12-Inch Solid Double Dong" — Guess they needed a name as long as the box. Jel material is all the rage in dildos and vibrators right now. It's soft and rubbery, but still firm. This particular dildo has the interesting design of a penis shape at both ends. If you're going solo, you could use it for vaginal and anal penetration at the same time, which, I imagine, would provide some novel sensations. If you're with a partner, you could try other combinations, like one end in his anus and the other in yours, or in your vagina, or vagina to vagina. It has all sorts of obscene possibilities. Also makes a great rolling-pin for strudel. ✳✳

"Natural Contours" — Another hot item with the ladies on the crew. It's a vibrator, curved so it fits in your hand, and looks more like a lady's shaver than a sex device. Great for travelling. In fact, Sue carries one in her car, but not for the reason you think. Here's her excuse:

"This chartreuse jobbie certainly caught our attention. 'Natural Contours' has a futuristic shape and design. This vibrator is not for penetration, but for genital stimulation of both males and females. It's also good for stiff shoulders during a long drive. The kids will never know what its primary purpose is, but your partner will get the message, and the massage, loud and clear." ★★★★

"Butt Really" — We get many questions about anal intercourse from both women and men, and this is the device we recommend for first-timers. It's a simple vibrator that consists of a thin, rubber, five-inch dildo powered by a removable, vibrating bullet. Since it's no wider than a middle finger, insertion is painless. The rubber is firm but flexible, and it easily reaches a male's "A" spot for orgasmic stimulation. It's a bonus that you can actually boil the dildo section in water to clean it. Martha Stewart would approve. ★★★★

"Rubba Duckie" — Water-related toys are another trend in the sex gizmo market. These are designed primarily for women who like to cap off a soothing, hot, bubble bath with some masturbatory fun. The "Shower Massage" has been getting a bit stale, but never fear — "Rubba Duckie" has landed. This vibrator, cleverly disguised as a bathtub toy, is waterproof and floats. The kids can even play with it. But when you turn it on, that soft, rubber, vibrating beak will return the favour. Soon you'll be quacking for more. This is one of Sue's favourites, mainly for its sheer inventiveness. ★★★

"Artificial Vagina" — An interesting variation on a vibrator, this has an inflatable, rubber sleeve into which a male inserts his penis and adjusts the tightness by increasing the pressure. Here is Sue's review:

"Guys, you are never stuck with this sex toy. Some lubricant and a sexual fantasy and you're off. Use some manual stimulation to start the process, then place the penis in the open end, pump up the pressure for a comfortable grip, and adjust the vibrations. Wearing a condom makes mopping up easier. For a male who has the idea that he needs intercourse to be satisfied, this toy takes the pressure off his partner if she is just not in the mood for a passionate connection."

Sue also noted that the device was small enough that businessmen could travel with one of these in their briefcase, which forever changed the way that Julie looks at men in airports. **

"Squirmy Dragon" (a.k.a. "Rabbit Pearl") — This is the only time I saw the women fight over a vibrator. I won't tell you who won. Apparently, it's amazing. Here's what Sue had to say:

"It is usually called the 'Rabbit Pearl,' but this one is the 'Squirmy Dragon.' It's a long translucent, white and mauve vibrator that rotates and has little pearl beads enclosed in the shaft. Then, there is a fairly firm purple dragon that protrudes near the base. This lights up brilliant red and vibrates to stimulate the clitoris during penetration. The control, which is located in the base, allows you to vary the speed and direction of the rotating head."

From what I'm told, the rotating band of pearls inside of it offers a continuous, gentle massage to the vaginal walls. The sensations are overwhelming. ****

"Purple Venus Butterfly" — Another fave with the ladies on the crew. This is a vibrator that you actually wear, which has a certain advantage. Sue's comments:

"The 'Purple Venus Butterfly' is an imaginative device — a small vibrator shaped like a large butterfly. It is held in place by adjustable, elastic straps. The head of the butterfly provides clitoral stimulation and the body stimulates the vaginal opening, which is where all the nerve endings are located. The remote control provides more than enough stimulation, and it leaves your hands free to stimulate other parts of your body. Wow!" ***

"Ben Wah Balls" — An ancient and excellent sex toy. The voice of experience can wrap up this section:

"'Ben Wah Balls' come in a variety of sizes. Some are designed for insertion into the vagina where they provide gentle stimulation as you do the vacuuming or sit at the computer. The cord connecting the balls should be plastic, which is easy to wash and clean. Fabric cord is not a great idea. Some of the larger ones don't have cord. They are simply placed in the vagina. A word of warning — remove the heavier metal ones before you sit on the john. They could plop out and crack the bowl. Try to explain that to the plumber. There are 'Ben Wah Balls' for anal stimulation for men and women. Well lubricated, they may be inserted into the rectum during foreplay and sex. They provide increased prostatic stimulation that can be pleasurable. You gotta make sure the string does not get up into the rectum since that makes removal tricky. Be very relaxed during insertion and use lots and lots of water-based lubrication. Wash well after use and, as usual, do not share your toys." ****

The Top-Rated "Pleasure Chest": Models 'R' Us

"You know what I'd love to see?" Sue is leaning back in her chair, feet up on the boardroom table. "I'd love to see a men's lingerie show."

"Ah, great idea Sue," Julie stalls. We all wait for the inevitable next line. "How are we going to pay for it?" That's always a producer's response.

It's January 1999. We've just returned from Christmas break. Sue has obviously spent some of her vacation contemplating scantily-clad men as well as developing a plan to con Julie into this.

"Well, we could borrow some sexy outfits from a store, you know, leopard skin boxer shorts, that sort of thing, and I could make some skimpy outfits myself." Sue's working up a head of steam now. "You know, the firemen always put out a sexy calendar every year. Maybe we could get them to model for us. They'd probably do it for free just to promote the new calendar."

Julie likes that word, "free." She also likes thinking about firemen. "Hey, that's not a bad idea." The other two of us in the meeting — Shanda Deziel and I — watch the gears turning. "Maybe we could do it for Valentine's Day!" Score one point for Sue.

Having done a lot of fashion shoots, I pipe up. "We should probably pre-tape it. Sue will have to do a voice-over on top of it, and trying to co-ordinate all that and the models on a live show could be messy, especially at 11:30 at night."

Julie deflates. "Well, we really don't have it in the budget to do a field shoot." Penalty for Sue.

"We could just tape it here and use a studio camera," I suggest. "Shoot it in the hallway or on the staircase, before a show."

That goes over big. We're just about to dial 911 when Sue throws a curve ball.

"Why don't we ask the guys on the crew if they'll be the models?"

Time out. Silence. You could have heard an I.U.D. drop. Slowly, images start to form in everyone's imagination, and chuckles start to percolate up, like bubbles in a pot of porridge. It's a home run!

"Okay, that would be great, but I'm not asking them," I say. The thought of asking my male colleagues to prance around in their skivvies is just *too* embarrassing. "*You're* asking them."

"No problem. I'll ask them." And with that, Sue pushes herself away from the table, and marches off the playing field. Julie, Shanda, and I grin at each other, shrug our shoulders, and giggle. We are enjoying shared thoughts of average guys with average bodies trying to look like stud-muffins. None of us could have foreseen that Sue's scheme was going to develop into the most popular episode of the *Sunday Night Sex Show* that ever aired.

In the end, there were four crew members who volunteered for this dangerous assignment: Germain, Ivan, Derrick, and Dwayne. Ali shot the segment with a hand-held camera after Derrick worked out the lighting for shooting it on the staircase.

We all arrived early on a Sunday evening, including the women on the crew. There was no way they were going to miss this momentous occasion.

Sue handed over the costumes, and the guys began to look

bilious. She had picked up some red spandex shorts, a leopard skin jockstrap, boxer shorts with a tuxedo front, a royal-blue spandex bikini, and — the clincher — a G-string with googly eyes, floppy ears, and an elephant trunk on the front. We all knew which part of the anatomy the trunk was designed for.

Since it was close to Valentine's Day, there had been a sale on seasonal fabrics at her favourite store, Fabricland, so she'd beefed up the beefcake by sewing a few of the items herself — boxer shorts with silver hearts all over them, a matching black-silk smoking jacket, and a leopard-skin sarong to go with the jockstrap.

"Okay fellas," she said cheerfully. "Who's going to wear what?" Judging by their reaction, she may as well have asked who wanted a cavity search. She quickly realized she was going to have to help this along.

"Dwayne, why don't you wear the boxer shorts with hearts with this black smoking jacket over it?"

That sounded safe. Everyone's sphincter relaxed, and suddenly, our models turned into a giggly gaggle of schoolboys. They disappeared into the dressing room, spandex in tow. Out in the hallway, all we heard was guffawing and chortling, punctuated by the occasional "No way!"

Now, you have to understand how much courage it takes to do something like this. Neither Ali nor I had the guts to do it. With the exception of Germain, who has the hard body of a professional wrestler, most of us on the show have generic, middle-class bodies at best. No sculpted abs or bulging baskets here. Consider that the average male is skittish about modelling his new down-filled, Eddie Bauer winter coat in front of his wife. These guys were going to appear on national television with only a thin layer of fabric between them and public humiliation.

Finally, they emerged, looking a tad sheepish. One of them took me aside, Dwayne I think, and said, "We'd like to do this without the women standing around watching. Could you ask them to go to the Control Room?"

"Sure," I responded. "Ladies, we would appreciate it if you would watch the shoot from the Control Room," I announced. "The guys would feel more comfortable, if you don't mind."

Julie, Sana, Liisa, Liz, and Shanda unhappily trudged away down the corridor, disappearing from view. Sue wanted to make some last minute adjustments to the apparel. There was one thing in particular that wasn't looking quite right.

"There was one outfit that needed to be padded out in the front," she explains delicately, "so I went into the women's washroom to get some toilet paper. That was where it struck me — why not an empty toilet paper tube? There was one sitting there, so I grabbed it."

Yes, if the truth be told, one of the guys from that famous episode had a toilet paper tube chunking up his natural assets. That model shall remain nameless, but it should be pointed out that the garment in question appeared to have been designed for the "dangly bits" of a sperm whale, not a human male.

Then I came within a pubic hair's breadth of making matters even more embarrassing. He had placed his penis inside the tube, and then the tube inside his garment. Well, it still looked like a toilet paper tube poking against the tight fabric, so, being the director, I thought, "Well, if I just crush it that will get rid of the round contours on the ends." I was just reaching for it when a voice in my head shouted, "Holy shit, his dick's in there!" and my open hand came to an abrupt halt a scant centimetre away from his genitals. "Can you just crush it a bit?" I suggested gingerly. That solved the problem.

We positioned the camera at the foot of the stairs, and each model came down one at a time. To our astonishment, they were absolutely awesome. Each guy strutted his stuff without a hint of self-consciousness, twirling on the landing, flashing a thumb's up at the camera. Derrick breezed down the stairs, looking very coy in the tuxedo boxer shorts. Dwayne, puffing on a cigar, did an elaborate striptease, slowly opening his smoking jacket, revealing the boxer shorts, turning and shaking his booty. Ivan chose the tight, red, spandex shorts and when he spun around, we quickly understood why. Who knew he had a bubble-butt? He spun it to the camera and gave it a nasty slap. And Germain — well, he may as well have been naked. First he appeared wearing the sarong, which he removed to reveal leopard skin shorts. Then he tantalizingly lowered these to display the leopard skin jockstrap. It was very sultry and sexy. But, when he showed up the second time wearing the elephant-front G-string, there was just about nothing left to the imagination. He did a slow turn to reveal the back, which was non-existent except for the black, elastic band around his waist. That's right — a fully naked, hunky butt-shot on the *Sunday Night Sex Show*. If the Grey Nuns had been watching, they would have stampeded to the confessionals.

While the guys were preoccupied with the task at hand, the women were having a virtual "Stag-ette party" in the Control Room. We later discovered that they were watching the proceedings on all the monitors, with much hooting, hollering, and occasional moaning. In fact, they were making so much noise that they had to close the Control Room door.

"Oh my God. Check out Ivan's ass!" (Hoot. Hoot. Hoot.)

"Oh, Derrick is soooo cute. Don't you just want to take him home!" (Group sigh.)

"Dwayne is just so cool. Ha! Look at that wiggle!" (Hoot. Hoot. Hoot.)

"Germain, Germain, Germain — be still my beating heart!" (Group lubrication.)

"Is it getting hot in here, or is it just me?"

"We had such a riot!" says Liisa. "In most jobs, you don't get to see your co-workers wearing practically nothing, and we couldn't believe that these guys we'd been working with for years were hiding these bodies under their clothes. And they were just so brave. They looked so confident and relaxed."

When the segment aired, WTN was flooded with calls from viewers who loved it. One call they didn't get was from Germain's mother, who was less than impressed. She let her son know that she didn't approve at all of him flaunting his assets on national television.

In the meantime, in case you missed our comrades being steamy, here's Sue's commentary with stills from the notorious men's lingerie shoot:

Ladies, how could you resist Derrick in these spectacular leopard shorts? Not subtle, these shorts demand immediate attention. Looks so good, bet you can't wait to get into them. Purrrrr . . .

What a well dressed man wears when he goes formal. Derrick wears these Tuxedo boxer shorts, complete with stud buttons for the big stud inside. Don't you just wish this gorgeous guy came with the shorts? (Fig. 1)

Our own Ivan sports these smashing red spandex shorts accented with slinky nylon black lace inserts. These revealing but concealing shorts put a whole new meaning to "Stay cool man . . ." (Fig. 2)

Germain covers up with the animal pattern sarong for men. A quick jerk and the Velcro tab releases to reveal these luxurious black shorts with leopard inserts. But whoa, what have we got here?! Naughty, naughty, naughty. (Fig. 3)

Dwayne gets in the mood with this sophisticated smoking jacket with a leopard on the back to display the animal in him. This cover up will not give away your secret desire to make mad passionate love. . . . It is what's under the jacket, those silver hearts and that sexy wiggle. (Fig. 4)

Here we see Ivan wearing these sparkling, royal blue, spandex exercise shorts. He's ready for the best 20-minute workout in bed.

There's a bit of red fluff but the eyes have it. . . . Like Pinocchio, the nose cone gets larger as the evening goes on, so there is no doubt what your intentions are. Strictly honourable, of course. Germain is our hot model for this steamy number.

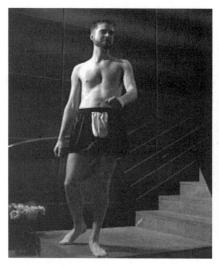

FIGURE 1

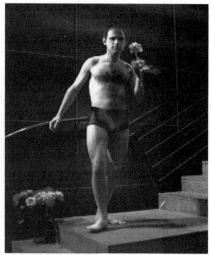

FIGURE 2

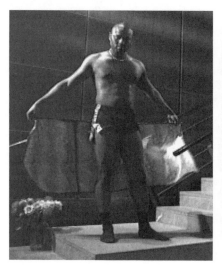

FIGURE 3

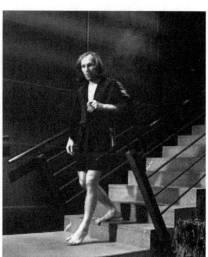

FIGURE 4

In subsequent seasons, we tried to organize a women's lingerie shoot with the ladies on the crew, but it has never panned out. It's the difference in gender power and politics. When men strip, it's just fun — when women strip, it's a come-on. Men don't feel threatened walking around in their underwear, whereas women do. Nevertheless, some of the ladies are gung-ho, so don't be surprised if you tune in one night and see "Models 'R' Us — Part Two."

"Myth-Conceptions" Quiz

Going into our fourth season, Sue suggested that we do a bumper on each show that presented a common sexual myth. We decided to title it "Myth-Conception" and developed it into a mini-quiz with a "True" or "Myth" answer.

We would always pre-tape this bumper and flash the correct answer under the question. Adrian Hepes, a Romanian who was our technical producer at the time, was quite incapable of saying "myth." To the Control Room's great delight, he would shout out "Mitt, Mitt" if he thought the statement was false. This became the running gag, and we would never package the bumper without Adrian in the room. It became such a signature moment that, after he left the show, we dropped the bumper. (Well, we were running out of myths anyway.)

So, here's your chance to yell out "Mitt, Mitt" in the privacy of your own home. You may want to warn other residents and your canary before proceeding. If you're Romanian, this won't be much of a challenge.

Here are Sue's "Myth-Conceptions" and here's the twist — only one of these is "True." Can you find it?

1. If you swallow ejaculate, it will give you big breasts, clear up your acne, and eliminate your menstrual cramps.
2. Homosexuals always have strong mothers and weak fathers.
3. Not every female has a G-spot.
4. Sexual education promotes early sexual activity.
5. Pulling out is a good method of birth control.
6. Guys are hornier than girls.
7. If you masturbate, you will have a reduced sperm count.

8. You can't have sex while you are pregnant because it will harm the baby.
9. You can get a sexually transmitted disease from a toilet seat.
10. A guy can get trapped in a vagina.
11. If you have had a heart attack, you cannot have sex.
12. It takes women longer to climax than men.
13. You can't get pregnant if you're breastfeeding.
14. It always hurts the first time you have sex.
15. You can't have sex during your period.
16. Gay men have larger penises than straight men.
17. A penis pump will make the penis larger.
18. Brunettes taste better than blondes.
19. Spanish Fly is an aphrodisiac.
20. Nice girls don't carry condoms.
21. A man can always tell if a woman is faking an orgasm.
22. You can't get pregnant the first time you have sex.

Sorry to tell you, fellas, but number sixteen is true. No one has any idea why this occurs, but on average, gay men have larger penises than heterosexual men. They also have a higher than average I.Q., which probably confirms women's oft-stated belief that a guy's brains are in his dick.

Cross-Country Croquet

"You expect us to shoot the ball through *that?!*" Frances protests, looking at Dwayne and me.

"Well, it's a bit of a challenge," Dwayne earnestly responds, "but we tried it, and you can do it." He adds, with a shrug, "Might take you a couple of shots."

This is one of the most diabolical traps he has yet devised. He's placed the white croquet hoop about a foot away from a bundle-buggy, and placed an upside-down shovel on the ground in front of the buggy. The idea is to use the inverted scoop of the shovel as a ramp to launch the croquet ball through the rungs of the bundle-buggy, and have it go through the hoop on the other side.

I try to encourage Frances. "I did it in practice before we started, and it works. The ball actually landed inside the bundle-buggy, and then I just knocked it out from there."

"Harrumph," she snorts. We receive a withering glance, and then she focuses on the

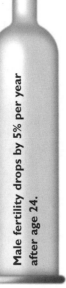

Male fertility drops by 5% per year after age 24.

blue, wooden ball at her feet. Her partner, Julie, urges her on.

"Frances, you can do it. Just take your time."

Dwayne is the principal engineer of our annual cross-country croquet game, staged at Sue's cottage each summer. She owns a large property on Lake Simcoe, about an hour and a half north of Toronto, and many crew members make the trek for this event. In fact, some have turned down other work to be here. An afternoon of swimming, croquet, yapping, barbecue, and free booze — it's hard to say no. It's the perfect spot, since there are actually two separate cottages on the site, and nearly everyone stays over for brunch the next morning.

Frances whacks the ball straight on. It shoots up the shovel, sails through the rungs of the buggy, and lands directly beside the hoop.

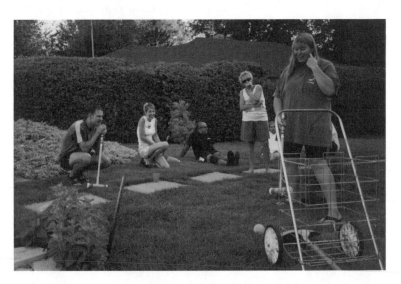

Liz confronts the bundle buggy trap while Ivan, Liisa, Sue, and Dwayne anticipate the approaching disaster. Ali is looking for fish.

"Yeah!" Julie shouts. "Thank God I've got you for a partner!" Frances takes a bow.

"Yeah," says Ali, with slightly less enthusiasm as he surveys the shot from a prone position. It's been several beers and his grasp of the game's complexities is approaching "zero miles an hour." He and his drinking partner, Ivan, are far back in the field, stymied by a trap of Ivan's own demented imagination — a hoop on top of a stump. The rest of us had cleared it, but those two, with their red ball, were having a hell of a time. Lying in the grass seemed like the best way to proceed.

"Zero miles an hour" is a _Sunday Night Sex Show_ catchphrase. It came from a strange call Sue received, several years ago, from a guy whose sexual fantasy was to have a woman rub her feet all over his face while they were driving "really, really slowwwwww, like zero miles an hour." We all agreed that that would be _very_ slow indeed, and snatched his memorable phrase for our own devious dialect.

"Who's next?" Liisa asks.

Dwayne checks the colours on his mallet. "Yellow. Sue and Liz."

"Am I up or are you?" Sue asks her partner.

"I think it's me," says Liz, stepping up to the yellow ball. They're coming up to the bundle-buggy, but have to clear a newly-planted forsythia bush first.

We've got five teams of two for this year's match: Frances and Julie, Sue and Liz, Dwayne and Derrick, Liisa and I, and Ali and Ivan. Sana is at home with her new baby boy and Germain is off wrestling in the Maritimes. Otherwise, they would both be here for the festivities. They hate to miss a

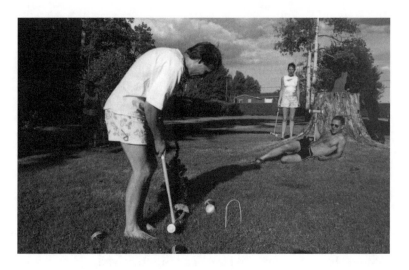

Dwayne plays with other people's balls while Liisa and Ivan anticipate the action.

good party. Of course, the arrival of the tornado at last year's event could hardly be topped.

On that occasion, it was a hot, sticky July afternoon and we were in the throes of the game. Gazing across the water, I saw a dark cloud gathering over the opposite shore of Lake Simcoe.

"That's a thunderhead," I announced, with all the authority of someone who has watched far too many weather specials on TLC. A preoccupation with weather seems to be an early sign of ageing. The cloud continued to grow as we played, blossoming upwards into the shape of an ominous, black mushroom. It drew closer to us. We dropped our mallets and headed indoors for supper. The cloud took on a tubular shape. A terrible rain started, a downpour jetting sideways, pushed by gale-force winds. As I gazed out the window, I knew that Peter

Coyote's authoritative narration would start at any moment.

"The hapless crew of a Canadian television program saw the storm coming, and did nothing. With the type of smugness only achieved through years of journalistic impertinence, they ignored the warning signs until it was too late. Their crumpled bodies were later discovered in the rubble, bludgeoned by croquet balls and blunt sexual devices. It was a tragic reminder of the awesome power of nature . . ."

Suddenly, my reverie was interrupted by Liisa screaming at me.

"Randy! Sue's run outside. She's running over to the other cottage. Stop her!"

I turned to the window just in time to see Sue staggering down the path, fighting the wind and the rain, as branches, leaves, and the odd guinea fowl, swirled by. She was totally nuts, and Liisa was even crazier if she thought I was going to run out there, too. Sue had gotten it into her head that she had better shut the windows in the other cottage. Apparently, being sucked up by a tornado was far less troublesome than having wet floors.

She made it to the other building and stayed there until the storm passed. The tornado hit just south of us, devastating two farms in the process. When we emerged to retrieve our fearless host, Mother Nature offered a compensation for her disruptive behaviour — a glorious double-rainbow formed overhead. None of us had ever seen such a thing. We "ooh'd" like little children standing under a vast Christmas tree. Now, how can you beat a party like that?

Thwack! Liz has taken a novel approach to the obstacle at hand, although a croquet mallet is not generally considered a garden tool. The forsythia bush folds in two as the yellow ball cuts through it (lopping the top off), bounces off the metal shovel with a 'ping,' and disappears into the cedar hedge.

"Oh, shit. Sorry Sue. I guess I hit it too hard."

Sue is laughing. "No problem. It'll grow back. The problem is I have to make the next damn shot!" They wander off to find the wayward missile.

"We're up," says Derrick, poised over the orange ball. He's such a gentle person that you can't imagine he'll have the heart to hit it. In the studio, Derrick is Sue's touchstone. She says that when she looks up and sees him behind the camera, she knows everything is right with the world. "I get such a sense of comfort and acceptance from both him and Germain," she says.

When he was a teenager, Derrick and his friends would sit in a car in a parking lot so that they could listen to Sue's show on the radio, unfettered by parental disapproval. It was their Sunday night rebellion. He could never have predicted that, one day, he'd be hanging out at her cottage.

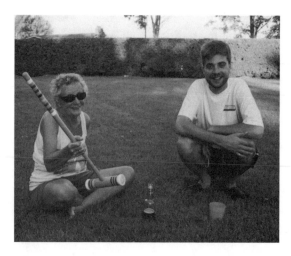

Sue and Derrick
share a beer.

"I guess I expected Sue to be just another host," he says. "Camera guys are taught not to talk to the host or guests, but she was friendly right away. She didn't have that TV attitude and was not self-important." He glances over at her butt sticking out of the hedge. "She's like a grandmother, and she has age and wisdom that I don't have. Relating to her is like relating to a friend. To me, she seems like she's 25."

Dwayne eyes his partner. "Just tap it into a good position, okay?" He's getting anxious to tackle the bundle-buggy.

"Okay, okay," Derrick responds. He gives the ball a gentle knock and it lands at the base of the shovel. "There. Set you up."

"Ha! You set us up, too," I point out. Liisa and I are next and the orange ball is right in our path. According to the very strict, internationally sanctioned, highly official, virtually inarguable, approved by the Synod of Bishops "Cross-Country Croquet" rules, we just need to touch their ball and we get an extra turn. We confer:

"Just roll up and tap their ball and that will leave us at the base of the shovel and then we can knock it through." "Right, but not too hard. We could knock their ball out but then we'd miss the shovel." "Right." Oh, the strategies. This game makes polo look downright wussy.

It's Liisa's shot, and she stands directly over our green ball to line it up. Her determination is palpable. It's the same indefatigable will she displays when she's helping to organize the Christmas dinner.

The _Sunday Night Sex Show_ always takes two weeks off over Christmas out of deference to those who feel that sex and religiosity are non-compatible. No edible panties under the tree

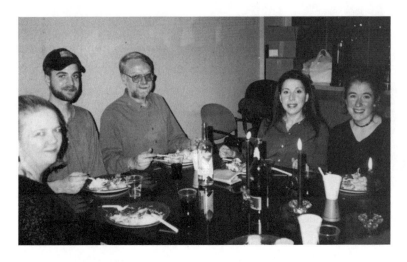

*The Christmas potluck dinner: Julie, Derrick, RJ, Sana, and Lynda.
Check out the candles!*

for them! We are happy to have the break. On the last Sunday before we go, our other great "family" tradition has evolved — the Christmas potluck dinner. Liisa is a major proponent.

We come in early before the show and crowd into the boardroom for our feast. Because of the diverse ethnicity of the crew, it's potluck with an international flair. Sana brings *shawarma*, an Arab dish; Sue makes individual meat pies and sourdough biscuits; Priya makes homemade *roti*; Dwayne brings his wife Christine's amazing "Heavenly Salad"; Ali brings an Iranian dish prepared by his mother; Julie bakes a chocolate-pecan pie; Liz makes a spectacular seven-layer dip; Lynda brings a Maltese dish, *pastizzi*; and on and on. WTN provides the wine (which is consumed sparingly, since we have a live show to do) and the table is set with candles and festive centrepieces. The food is arrayed on the wide window-ledge in a long, multi-national smorgasbord, and we dig in. Of course, by the time we're done, we all want to fall asleep. In fact, one year, Sue _did_ fall asleep just outside the studio door while resting in a comfy armchair. Luckily, Sana discovered her before the show or it would have been Germain fielding questions for an hour. ("Germain, do you know any other sexual positions besides a 'half-Nelson'?")

When people hedge about the Christmas dinner because it's so much work, Liisa is its most ardent advocate. "Where else do you get a chance to taste all those different flavours from around the world?" she argues. Everyone relents and this disparate blend of atheists, agnostics, Christians, Muslims, and Hindus share a jolly Christmas meal together.

Tap! Liisa has just kissed the orange ball with ours.

I say, "Good. Now just whack it through the buggy."

"I'll try." She takes aim and shoots from the side, hitting it hard. The ball sails up the shovel ramp, dings on a rung, and lands directly inside the bundle-buggy.

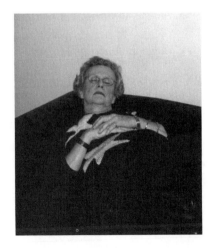

Yes, 10 minutes to air and the host is fast asleep in the hallway outside the studio door. (Photo courtesy Sana Natur)

"Fuck!" she yelps. She used to be so much more proper.

"Hey, no problem. I'll just scoop it out on my shot. Who's up next?" I ask. Everyone checks the mallet handle for the line-up.

"Red!" "Red!" "It's red!" "Red!"

We all look back at Ivan and Ali. They are both lying on the ground by the stump, looking up at the clouds.

"Do you see that fish up there?" Ali is pointing at the sky. "There's a huge fucking fish up there. Looks like a salmon."

Ivan considers it. "More like a pickerel."

"Red, it's your turn!"

They struggle to their feet. "Look guys," says Ali, in his most earnest tone, "we've taken three turns trying to get through this hoop. I think three should be the limit and then you move on automatically."

The rest of us consider their request. Since the Synod isn't in session, and since they're so far behind they don't have a hope in hell of winning anyway, we agree to let them off the hook. Suddenly the fish allusion becomes clear.

Ali sets their ball in front of the bundle-buggy, and then takes a characteristically novel approach. He lies face down in the grass and takes aim with the handle of his mallet, using it as a pool cue. Now, there is a possibility that standing is not an option at this point, but we are all familiar with how Ali's mind works. After all, we'd seen him with a "Thigh Rider" attached to his forehead for an entire evening.

The "Thigh Rider" is a long, black, rubber dildo with a strap on it. It's designed for paraplegics or quadriplegics, and one uses it by tying it to one's thigh. The dildo sticks straight up, and one's partner rides it for sexual stimulation.

188

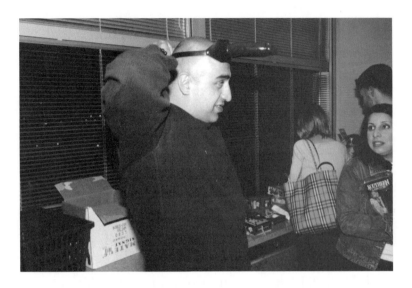

Ali tries on "The Thigh Rider," although he missed the intended anatomical locale. Sana considers his sanity.

At the end of each television season, Sue brings in most of the sex toys she's accumulated throughout the year (she *does* keep some herself), and we have our annual "Sex Toy Scramble." At first, Julie thought people would be too demure to lunge for dildos, and envisioned a more discreet session where we would each enter the boardroom alone and politely choose our "tools." No way. The entire assemblage descends en masse, jostling and shoving each other, lobbing vibrators back and forth, and shooting cock-rings like rubber bands off the boardroom walls. It's like staging the Hadassah Bazaar at the Playboy mansion.

"Hey Sana, do you want this 'Squirmy Dragon'?"

"Germain, you'd look great in this 'Adonis Pouch'!"

"Sue, where's the 'Fukuoku'?"

"At home, honey!"

"You should take the 'Blue Angel.' It matches your eyes."

"Does this come with batteries?"

"I don't know. Do _you_ come with batteries?"

"Do you think these vibrating panties will fit me?"

"Probably, but what will your wife say?"

"'Deep Penetrating Dong,' anyone?"

I know where only three of the toys ended up: Liisa got the
"Ben-Wah Balls," which she gave to her boyfriend's cat; Ali
strapped the "Thigh Rider" to his forehead and wore it
throughout the show (and probably all the way home); and I
took "Auto Jill," strictly out of pity, mind you. Nobody else
wanted her. Working on the _Sunday Night Sex Show_ is one of
the few jobs where you get a boner instead of a bonus at the
end of the year.

Now, it may seem odd to an outsider that we're so casual
about sex toys and our personal preferences, but it's an occu-
pational hazard — or merit — in this case. That attitude of
being supportive and non-judgmental simply filters down
from the host. As Shanda Deziel observed, "I guess that's part
of why we have to be a family. If we weren't all close, how
could we look at each other while this stuff is going on all
around us? For me to go into that studio and play with vibrators as Ali sat in the corner typing, I had to feel like I could do
anything in front of him."

Boink. The red ball rolls up the shovel, off the side of it,
and under the buggy.

Ali drops his face into the lawn. "Fuck," he mutters.

Ultimately, Frances and Julie prevailed. They won the match

and then headed for the cottage kitchen to make hamburgers for the barbecue. Since I was the first man to get through the course, I was consigned to cooking. Barbecues are generally the realm of men, presumably because they're outside, which is where women prefer us. We can guard against sabre-toothed tiger attacks _and_ do something domestic at the same time. The same principle applies to taking the garbage out and cleaning eavestroughs. This strategy works brilliantly — a sabre-toothed tiger has never been spotted in our neighbourhood. Raccoons, however, are impervious to this show of virility.

We ate on Sue's deck and continued laughing and chattering long after darkness had fallen. People talked of the difficult game, cursing Dwayne. We talked about favourite moments of the past season, poking fun at each other, annoying each other, trumpeting each other, and sharing the mirth together. It was the three A's in full bloom — acceptance, acknowledgement, and appreciation. Finally, Sue and I retired to her place, and the gang settled into the other, larger cottage.

As I waited for her to brush her teeth in the bathroom, I gazed across the lawn at the other building. A single light gleamed from the living room, glinting off the dew on the grass. I knew they were still yapping away over there. It reminded me of the signature closing of _The Waltons_, when the family members wrapped up the episode with a voice-over and then said goodnight. Yeah, it was sappy, but it had a sweet simplicity about it that always rang true. Sana's words from the interview I had done with her came back to me:

"We're so tight. We're just a really close crew. I think that we accept each other no matter what. We're genuinely family because, even if we don't love every single thing about each other, we learn to tolerate everything because, you know what, we're stuck with each other. That's family, and that's it."

"What a glorious day," says Sue, joining me at the window. She sighs. "I love those guys."

And with that, she turns and trundles off to her room, weary with pleasure. I close the blind for the night. The light next door is still on.

While doing research for this book, I read through many scripts of past episodes of the Sunday Night Sex Show. *Herbal remedies for ailments involving the reproductive system popped up repeatedly. So, I asked Sue Johanson if she would compile the various bits of information into a brief chapter, and she kindly agreed. She also included instructions for Kegel exercises, another topic we are often asked about. Take it away, Sue!*

Women who consume the caffeine in 3 cups of coffee or 8 soft drinks per day reduce their monthly chance of conceiving by 26%.

Sexual Health and Herbs
By Sue Johanson

Menopause Naturally

At about age 45, many women start experiencing symptoms of *perimenopause,* that 10-year span before your menstrual periods actually stop. One year without a period and you are officially "menopausal."

Anatomically, your ovaries are ageing, becoming old and wrinkled. They do not release an egg every month, although you still have periods. There will also be a slight decline in the production of testosterone.

Outward signs and symptoms include night sweats, hot flashes, dry skin, and the appearance of wrinkles. The flesh at the back of your arms and thighs starts to feel loose and floppy, your breasts lose their "oomph," and your waist becomes thicker as more fat is deposited on your abdomen. Your libido may be reduced. Some women experience heart palpitations.

Moods may swing from gloriously happy to depressed, confused, angry, and accusatory. You may cry for no apparent reason. You may be forgetful: unable to find the right word or constantly losing your keys. These are sometimes called "menopause moments." Personally, I prefer to call them "brain farts."

Less obvious body changes include vaginal dryness; decreased lubrication may make intercourse uncomfortable. Also, the mucous membrane lining of the vagina thins out, so you get little abrasions with ordinary sex and sex may be painful. You may notice that you dribble urine when you laugh, cough, or sneeze; and when you "gotta go," you gotta go NOW or you are in trouble. Before you buy a package of Attends, start doing Kegel exercises. They really do work if you do them regularly and frequently. A description of Kegel exercises is coming up shortly.

Unbeknownst to you, there may be calcium coming out of your bones, leaving them brittle and porous so that they break easily, especially your hips and spine. Called *osteoporosis*, this may lead to what is called "widow's hump," those hunched over, rounded shoulders. Osteoporosis is serious. It seems to affect white women, fair skinned, blue eyed, and slight or slender women.

Does this sound familiar? Well, your doctor may want you

to consider "Hormone Replacement Therapy" (HRT). But, your friends may be talking about "natural" menopause, using nutrition and herbal supplements.

This is not as easy as it sounds. You are going to have to alter your diet, reduce sugars, coffee, tea, and colas. You'll need to take in more fibre and many more fresh fruits and vegetables. You'll need less carbohydrates and less red meat. Soy, found in tofu or soy milk, has a mild estrogenic effect, but it takes a lot of soy to meet your needs.

There are a few brands of supplements sold as a "complex" which are supposed to contain all the necessary herbal supplements, but there are warnings that they may not be as "complete" as they are cracked up to be. Not enough research has been done, and there have been no long-term studies.

Here is a list of the herbal supplements that have been recommended to prevent some of the side effects of menopause without resorting to HRT. The list is long. You will have to divide your medications so you are taking them at intervals during the day. As always, check with your doctor first. These are the daily dosages:

- Black Cohosh — 250 mg daily — supposed to calm nerves, improve pelvic muscle tone — may cause headache and nausea.
- Vitamin E — 800 iu daily — for hot flashes.
- Calcium — 1200 mg daily — avoid calcium carbonate which does not absorb well.
- Evening Primrose Oil — 1000 iu — essential fatty acid for hair and skin.
- B Complex Vitamin Supplement — containing Thiamin, Niacin, B6, B12, and Folic Acid.

- Vitamin C — 1000 mg.
- Vitamin D — for stronger bones — improves nervous system.
- Magnesium — for stronger bones, teeth, and muscles.
- Iron — improves blood circulation, muscle function, oxygen carrying power.
- Vitamin K — for blood clotting and regulation of calcium levels.
- Selenium — 100 mcg daily — boosts immune system.
- Beta Carotene — 25,000 iu.
- Zinc — 15 mg of either zinc citrate or picolate.
- Coenzyme Q10 — anti-oxidant — boosts immune system.
- Gingko Biloba — 120 mg — for cognitive functions, depression, migraines.
- Ginseng — 1000 to 2000 mg — combats toxins — improves oxygen supply to muscles.
- St. John's Wort — 300 mg — for depression.
- Valerian — helps relieve stress, aids sleep, and reduces muscle tension.
- Dong Quai — helps relieve symptoms of perimenopause and menopause.

Exercise is essential. Walking (foot to ground exercise) helps maintain bone density and prevent osteoporosis. It also helps eliminate fat and increase lean muscle mass.

Did you know that the female metabolism slows down by two percent per year starting in middle age? And did you know that women who smoke have about 25% less bone mass than those who don't? Keep those facts in mind.

Herbal and Nutritional Supplements — Other Problems

Please be advised that clinical studies on herbal remedies are lacking. Some herbal remedies may interfere with other drugs you may be using, or with other medical conditions you may have. Check with your physician before taking any alternative treatments.

Menstrual Problems and P.M.S.

Daily dosages:

- Calcium — 500–1000 mg.
- Manganese — 2 mg.
- Niacin — 25–200 mg beginning seven days before period due.
- Vitamin B6 — 150–200 mg. Check with your doctor first.
- Vitamin C — 1000 mg.
- Iron — 15 mg if periods are heavy.
- Ginseng.
- Wild Yam supplement from health food store.
- Black Cohosh supplement from health food store.
- Vitamin E — 400 iu.

Do not take Gingko Biloba if you are pregnant.

Prostate

These herbs and vitamins are for the treatment of *benign prostatic hyperplasia* (BPH), a common enlargement of the prostate in mature males. However, prostate problems could indicate a more serious ailment, so always check with your doctor first. Anecdotal evidence suggests that daily treatment with the following items helps to reduce the enlarged prostate in cases of BPH:

- Saw Palmetto supplement from health food store.
- Zinc — 160 mg in two divided doses.
- Beta Carotene — 15,000 iu.
- Magnesium — 400 mg.
- Selenium — 50–200 mcg
- Vitamin A — 10,000 iu.
- Vitamin B6 — 2 mg.
- Vitamin C — 1000–5000 mg.
- Vitamin E — 600 iu.

Impotence and Low Sex Drive

Again, anecdotal evidence indicates that daily intake of these supplements may be effective. Check with your doctor first.

- Zinc — 50 mg.
- Gingko Biloba — 40 mg.
- Saw Palmetto.
- Siberian Ginseng.
- L-Arginine.
- Glutamic Acid.
- L-Lysine.
- Puncture Vine — 750 mg.
- Hoary Goat Weed — 600 mg.
- Vitamin C — 1000–3000 mg.
- Vitamin E — 400–8000 iu.
- Borage Oil.
- Evening Primrose Oil — 1000 mg.

Wild Oats and Plumtree Berry extracts are said to increase testosterone levels.

Some herbal remedies may have adverse effects on male fertility.

Males who smoke a package of cigarettes a day for 20 years are four times as likely to be impotent.

Take Calcium Citrate for the best absorption of the supplement rather than Calcium Lactate or Calcium Gluconate.

Endometriosis

Endometriosis can be a debilitating and painful condition. Check with your doctor before starting this daily regimen.

- Beta Carotene — 25,000–50,000 iu.
- Biotin — 200 mg.
- Folic Acid — 400 mcg.
- Niacin — 50 mg.
- Pantothenic Acid — 50 mg.
- Riboflavin — 50 mg.
- Selenium — 25 mcg.
- Thiamin — 50 mg.
- Vitamin B6 and Vitamin B12 — 30–50 mg.
- Vitamin C — 1000–4000 mg.
- Vitamin E — 400–2000 iu.

Kegel Exercises

Kegel (kay-gel) exercises are a series of easy, no-sweat exercises that you can do anywhere, any time. Stuck in traffic, boring TV? Just start kegeling. You will not regret it, especially if you are pregnant or just had a baby, if you have had lower abdominal surgery, if you want to spice up your sex life. If you are a male who is experiencing erectile dysfunction (impotence), or if you simply want to "last longer," Kegels will also help.

Your pubococcygeal muscles act like a sling, suspended from your pubic bone in front to your coccyx or tailbone. These muscles support all your pelvic organs, bladder, uterus and bowel. Sphincters are rings of muscles that circle your rectum (anus), your bladder, and the vagina.

Muscle tone decreases as a result of pregnancy, surgery, menopause — or manopause — bladder infections, and simply ageing. You know the old expression, if you don't use it, you lose it.

So, you may laugh, cough, do aerobic exercises, and then spurt small amounts of urine. It's very embarrassing. Or you have been stuck in traffic, get home, put your key in the lock, and suddenly you gotta pee . . . *now*. . . . You crotch-clutch and dribble in your rush to the bathroom. You've got a problem.

Before you go to the doctor for treatment for incontinence, you can take charge. When you start to urinate, clamp down, tighten up, and try to stop the flow of urine. If you can't "cut it off," then you need to start/stop, start/stop every time you urinate.

Don't stop there. Here are some other exercises that are helpful:

Sit on a hard chair, lean forward, and tighten all your sphincter muscles, anal, vaginal, and urethral in succession, front to back. Hold the squeeze for one or two seconds, release, then contract from back to front.

If you are in a line-up at the store, you can squeeze all your pubococcygeal (PC) muscles and lift and tuck. You will notice that when you do this, you tuck in your tailbone and tighten your abdominal muscles at the same time. That's a good thing. Now, gradually, release the muscles, slowly, one by one.

Here's one they call the "Flutter." Contract and release all the PC muscles quickly and repeatedly.

All these exercises should be practised in sets of 10 times each, five times a day. As well, do the "start/stop" exercise every time you urinate.

There are many fringe benefits to Kegeling. Females will be able to tighten their vaginal muscles and grip their partner's penis more tightly, adding to their sexual pleasure. Partners will enjoy the sensation too.

Practising Kegels during pregnancy will reduce lower back pain, make delivery easier and faster, and will help prevent haemorrhoids. If the new mother starts Kegels shortly after delivery of the baby, her genitals will heal faster, she will regain vaginal sensitivity, and help prevent "sloppy vagina."

Kegels are not "just a girl thing." We know that there are no muscles in the penis, but males who practice Kegels improve muscle tone and strength; they also increase blood supply to their genitals, including their penis. The improved circulation will give firmer erections. Males who practise Kegels are also able to contract their PC muscles and delay ejaculation.

Most males envy women's ability to have multiple orgasms. Well, some men can do it too. Because they have trained themselves to contract their pubococcygeal muscles as they approach ejaculatory inevitability, they can have a "dry orgasm" without losing their erection. As this appears to be a learned skill, men who want to achieve multiple orgasms should practise when masturbating. Remember, "getting there is half the fun."

Think positive, think "PC muscles."

Condom Closers

Every episode of the *Sunday Night Sex Show* ends with a "Condom Closer," a humorous line from Sue that promotes safer sex. Most of these closers are created by Sue, but some come from students she meets at lectures and from the crew. So, it seems appropriate to let her have the last line of the show's story. Here are some of Sue's best "Condom Closers":

You won't get a goody 'til you wrap your woody.

Sex will be sweeter if you wrap your peter.

Don't be a loner; cover your boner.

Condoms: the pecker picker upper.

Condoms: the ups and downs, the ins and outs of great sex.

After you give that copulatory gaze, use a condom for lots of praise.

When in doubt, shroud your spout.

If you go into heat, package your meat.

Don't be a flake; cover your snake.

Don't be a dork; wrap your pork.

It don't take long to cover your schlong.

Condom and lube — get a package and tube.

Stop and think and then cover your dink.

Go for the safest tactic: wear a prophylactic.

When you hit the sack, wear a pecker pack.

Cover your dukie: use a touquie.

Wrap your wagger if you're going to shag her.

If it's gonna be a moaner, cover your boner.

When she's looking slinky, wrap your dinky.

Wrap your hose before it blows.

To stay in the pink, cover your dink.

Don't be a chump — cover your stump before you hump.

Before you wham bam, cover your ham.

Wrap your snake when you're on the make.

It only takes a jiffy to cover Mr. Stiffy.

If he's got 'pokey pants,' wear a condom before you dance.

Don't touch that bod 'til you've covered that rod.

Before you dip your wick, cover your dick.

Don't slip it in 'til you've covered your skin.